Subdural Hematomas

Editors

E. SANDER CONNOLLY Jr
GUY M. MCKHANN II

NEUROSURGERY
CLINICS OF NORTH AMERICA

www.neurosurgery.theclinics.com

Consulting Editors
RUSSELL LONSER
DANIEL K. RESNICK

April 2017 • Volume 28 • Number 2

ELSEVIER

1600 John F. Kennedy Boulevard • Suite 1800 • Philadelphia, Pennsylvania, 19103-2899

http://www.theclinics.com

NEUROSURGERY CLINICS OF NORTH AMERICA Volume 28, Number 2
April 2017 ISSN 1042-3680, ISBN-13: 978-0-323-52415-5

Editor: Stacy Eastman
Developmental Editor: Colleen Dietzler

Neurosurgery Clinics of North America (ISSN 1042-3680) is published quarterly by Elsevier Inc., 360 Park Avenue South, New York, NY 10010-1710. Months of issue are January, April, July, and October. Business and Editorial Offices: 1600 John F. Kennedy Blvd., Suite 1800, Philadelphia, PA 19103-2899. Customer Service Office: 11830 Westline Industrial Drive, St. Louis, MO 63146. Periodicals postage paid at New York, NY, and additional mailing offices. Subscription prices are $393.00 per year (US individuals), $665.00 per year (US institutions), $423.00 per year (Canadian individuals), $826.00 per year (Canadian institutions), $505.00 per year (international individuals), $826.00 per year (international institutions), $100.00 per year (US students), and $255.00 per year (international and Canadian students). International air speed delivery is included in all *Clinics* subscription prices. All prices are subject to change without notice. **POSTMASTER:** Send address changes to *Neurosurgery Clinics of North America*, Elsevier Periodicals Customer Service, 11830 Westline Industrial Drive, St. Louis, MO 63146. **Customer Service: 1-800-654-2452 (US and Canada). From outside the US and Canada, call: 1-314-453-7041. Fax: 1-314-453-5170. E-mail: JournalsCustomerService-usa@elsevier.com (for print support) and journalsonlinesupport-usa@elsevier.com (for online support).**

Reprints. For copies of 100 or more, of articles in this publication, please contact the Commercial Reprints Department, Elsevier Inc., 360 Park Avenue South, New York, NY 10010-1710. Tel. 212-633-3874; Fax: 212-633-3820; E-mail: reprints@elsevier.com.

Neurosurgery Clinics of North America is covered in *MEDLINE/PubMed (Index Medicus), EMBASE/Excerpta Medica, and Current Contents/Clinical Medicine (CC/CM).*

Contributors

CONSULTING EDITORS

RUSSELL LONSER, MD
Professor and Chair, Department of
Neurological Surgery, The Ohio State
University Wexner Medical Center,
Columbus, Ohio

DANIEL K. RESNICK, MD, MS
Professor and Vice Chairman, Program
Director, Department of Neurosurgery,
University of Wisconsin School of Medicine
and Public Health, Madison, Wisconsin

EDITORS

E. SANDER CONNOLLY Jr, MD
Bennett M. Stein Professor of Neurological
Surgery, College of Physicians and Surgeons,
Columbia University; New York Neurological
Institute, NY-Presbyterian Hospital, New York,
New York

GUY M. McKHANN II, MD
Associate Professor of Neurological Surgery,
College of Physicians and Surgeons, Columbia
University; New York Neurological Institute,
NY-Presbyterian Hospital, New York,
New York

AUTHORS

ISAAC JOSH ABECASSIS, MD
Resident Physician, Department of
Neurological Surgery, Harborview Medical
Center, University of Washington, Seattle,
Washington

FAWAZ AL-MUFTI, MD
Endovascular Surgical Neuroradiology
Program, Rutgers University-New Jersey
Medical School, Newark, New Jersey

GAVIN W. BRITZ, MD
Chairman, Department of Neurosurgery,
Houston Methodist Hospital, Houston, Texas

IAN A. BUCHANAN, MD
Department of Neurosurgery, Keck School of
Medicine, University of Southern California,
Los Angeles, California

JASON J. CARROLL, MD
Interventional Neuroradiology Fellow,
Department of Neurological Surgery,
Neurological Institute, New York Presbyterian
Hospital-Columbia University Medical Center,
New York, New York

JAN CLAASSEN, MD, PhD
Associate Professor of Neurology and
Neurosurgery, Department of Neurology,
Columbia University Medical Center,
New York, New York

VIRENDRA R. DESAI, MD
Resident Neurosurgery Physician, Department
of Neurosurgery, Houston Methodist Hospital,
Houston, Texas

M. SEAN GRADY, MD
Chairman and Charles Frazier Harrison
Professor of Neurosurgery, Department of
Neurosurgery, Hospital of the University of
Pennsylvania, Philadelphia, Pennsylvania

DAIPAYAN GUHA, MD
Division of Neurosurgery, Department of
Surgery, Toronto Western Hospital, University
of Toronto, Toronto, Ontario, Canada

JUDY HUANG, MD, FAANS
Professor, Program Director, Department
of Neurosurgery, Johns Hopkins University
School of Medicine, Baltimore, Maryland

LOUIS J. KIM, MD
Professor, Department of Neurological
Surgery, Harborview Medical Center;
Department of Radiology, University
of Washington, Seattle, Washington

SEAN D. LAVINE, MD
Associate Professor of Neurological Surgery
and Radiology, Department of Neurological
Surgery, Clinical Co-Director,
Neuroendovascular Services, Neurological
Institute, New York Presbyterian Hospital, New
York, New York; Director, Neurointerventional
Services, The Valley Hospital Ridgewood,
Ridgewood, New Jersey

KIWON LEE, MD, FACP, FAHA, FCCM
Associate Professor and Vice Chairman,
Department of Neurosurgery, McGovern
Medical School, University of Texas Health
Science Center at Houston, Houston, Texas

**R. LOCH MACDONALD, MD, PhD, FRCSC,
FAANS, FACS**
Division of Neurosurgery, Department of
Surgery, Toronto Western Hospital, University
of Toronto; Division of Neurosurgery, Keenan
Research Centre for Biomedical Science, Li Ka
Shing Knowledge Institute, St. Michael's
Hospital, Toronto, Ontario, Canada

WILLIAM J. MACK, MD
Department of Neurosurgery, Keck School of
Medicine, University of Southern California,
Los Angeles, California

STEPHAN A. MAYER, MD, FCCM
Chair, Department of Neurology, Henry Ford
Health System, Detroit, Michigan

PHILIP M. MEYERS, MD
Professor of Radiology and Neurological
Surgery, Department of Neurological Surgery,
Clinical Co-Director, Neuroendovascular
Services, Neurological Institute, Children's
Hospital of New York, New York Presbyterian
Hospital, New York, New York

MATTHEW PIAZZA, MD
Resident Neurosurgeon, Department of
Neurosurgery, Hospital of the University of
Pennsylvania, Philadelphia, Pennsylvania

JEREMY T. RAGLAND, MD
Assistant Professor, Departments of
Neurosurgery and Neurology, McGovern
Medical School, University of Texas
Health Science Center at Houston,
Houston, Texas

MICHAEL REZNIK, MD
Clinical Instructor, Department of Neurology,
Columbia University Medical Center,
New York, New York

DAVID ROH, MD
Assistant Professor, Department of Neurology,
Columbia University Medical Center,
New York, New York

ROBERT A. SCRANTON, MD
Resident Neurosurgery Physician, Department
of Neurosurgery, Houston Methodist Hospital,
Houston, Texas

ALEX B. VALADKA, MD
Professor and Chair, Department of
Neurosurgery, Virginia Commonwealth
University, Richmond, Virginia

RAFAEL A. VEGA, MD, PhD
Resident, Department of Neurosurgery,
Virginia Commonwealth University, Richmond,
Virginia

WUYANG YANG, MD, MS
Research Fellow, Department of Neurosurgery,
Johns Hopkins University School of Medicine,
Baltimore, Maryland

Contents

> The imaging of subdural hematoma has evolved significantly. Computed tomography and MRI have supplanted other procedures and rendered most obsolete for the evaluation of intracranial pathology because of ease of use, tremendous soft tissue resolution, safety, and availability. Noncontrast computed tomography has become the accepted standard of care for the initial evaluation of patients with suspected subdural hematoma because of widespread availability, rapid acquisition time, and noninvasive nature. MRI offers important features in determining potential secondary causes of subdural hematoma, such as dural-based neoplasms.

> This article discusses the epidemiology and natural history of chronic subdural hematoma (CSDH), a common disease prevalent in the elderly population. The incidence of CSDH ranges from 1.72 to 20.6 per 100,000 persons per year. Risk factors include advancing age, male gender, and antiplatelet or anticoagulant use. Clinical progression is separated into 3 distinct periods, including the initial traumatic event, the latency period, and the clinical presentation period. The recurrence of CSDH and nonsurgical predictive factors are described in detail to provide a comprehensive understanding of the outcome of this disease.

> Chronic subdural hematomas (cSDHs) that are asymptomatic or have minimal symptoms have become more prevalent, with an increased rate of detection with neuroimaging in the setting of an aging population and increasing use of anticoagulants. These cSDHs have been known to spontaneously resolve, and subsequent efforts have been made to study the role of nonoperative initial medical management strategies in these patients. Current and potential strategies for the medical management of cSDH are discussed.

> Chronic subdural hematomas are one of the most common clinical entities encountered in today's neurosurgical practices owing to an aging population and continued increases in life expectancy. Although there is a role for conservative management, surgical drainage remains the mainstay of current therapy. Regardless of the technique used for hematoma drainage, there is level I evidence to suggest that use of closed-system drainage during the perioperative period significantly decreases the likelihood for hematoma recurrence, length of hospital stay, and mortality.

Isaac Josh Abecassis and Louis J. Kim

Chronic subdural hematomas are commonly encountered pathologies in neurologic surgery. Primary management for a symptomatic lesion usually entails surgical intervention. There is controversy regarding ideal modality selection among twist drill craniostomy, bur hole craniostomy, and craniotomy. Variations of the craniotomy include a minicraniotomy (usually defined as 30–40 mm diameter), minicraniectomy, and with or without either a partial or full membranectomy. In addition to medical complications, potential surgical complications include recurrence, seizures, intraparenchymal hemorrhage, and infection. Prior studies are summarized as well as rates of mortality, morbidity, reaccumulation requiring repeat operation, and clinical outcomes.

Jeremy T. Ragland and Kiwon Lee

A chronic subdural hematoma (cSDH) is a collection of old blood products and blood breakdown products that have accumulated in the subdural space. cSDH is increasingly common due to the combination of more frequent use of anticoagulant and antiplatelet agents and the advanced age of the population. The incidence of cSDH is estimated to be between 3.4 and 58 per 100,000 person-years depending on the age of the population. The United Nations predicts that the percentage of the population above age 65 is expected to double between 2010 and 2050. cSDH is more prevalent in men, with a 3:1 male-to-female ratio.

Rafael A. Vega and Alex B. Valadka

Because published guidelines for surgical decision-making in patients with acute subdural hematomas (ASDHs) are based largely on case series and other weak evidence, management often must be individualized. Nonoperative management is a viable option in many cases. The literature is divided about the effects of anticoagulant and antiplatelet medications on rapid growth of ASDHs and on their likelihood of progression to large chronic subdural hematomas. Close clinical and radiologic follow-up is needed, both acutely to detect rapid expansion of an ASDH, and subacutely to detect formation of a large subacute or chronic subdural hematoma.

Matthew Piazza and M. Sean Grady

Cranioplasty following craniectomy for trauma is a common, safe neurosurgical procedure that restores the natural cosmesis and protective barrier of the skull and may be instrumental in normalizing cerebrospinal fluid dynamics after decompressive surgery. Understanding the factors influencing patient selection and timing of cranioplasty, the available materials and methods of skull reconstruction, and the technical nuances is critical for a successful outcome. Neurosurgeons must be prepared to manage the complications specific to this operation. This article reviews the indications, preoperative assessment and timing, most commonly used materials, operative technique, postoperative care, and complication management for cranioplasty.

Although urgent surgical hematoma evacuation is necessary for most patients with subdural hematoma (SDH), well-orchestrated, evidenced-based, multidisciplinary, postoperative critical care is essential to achieve the best possible outcome. Acute SDH complicates approximately 11% of mild to moderate traumatic brain injuries (TBIs) that require hospitalization, and approximately 20% of severe TBIs. Acute SDH usually is related to a clear traumatic event, but in some cases can occur spontaneously. Management of SDH in the setting of TBI typically conforms to the Advanced Trauma Life Support protocol with airway taking priority, and management breathing and circulation occurring in parallel rather than sequence.

Subdural hematomas commonly recur after surgical evacuation, at a rate of 2% to 37%. Risk factors for recurrence can be patient related, radiologic, or surgical. Patient-related risk factors include alcoholism, seizure disorders, coagulopathy, and history of ventriculoperitoneal shunt. Radiologic factors include poor brain reexpansion postoperatively, significant subdural air, greater midline shift, heterogeneous hematomas (layered or multi-loculated), and higher-density hematomas. Surgical factors include lack of or poor postoperative drainage. Most recurrent hematomas are managed successfully with burr hole craniostomies with postoperative closed-system drainage. Refractory hematomas may be managed with a variety of techniques, including craniotomy or subdural-peritoneal shunt placement.

Antiplatelet and anticoagulant drugs (antithrombotics) predispose to acute and chronic subdural hematomas. Patients on these drugs are at higher likelihood of presenting with larger hematomas and more severe neurologic deficits. Standard neurosurgical and neurocritical care of subdural hematomas involves reversal of antithrombosis preoperatively, whereas reversing antiplatelet drugs is less clear. This article highlights the spectrum of antithrombotic agents in common use, their mechanisms of action, and strategies for reversal.

NEUROSURGERY CLINICS OF NORTH AMERICA

Preface

Contemporary Management of Subdural Hematomas

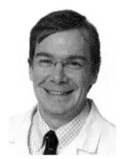 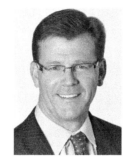

E. Sander Connolly Jr, MD   Guy M. McKhann II, MD
Editors

Given increased life expectancy, increased activity into older age, and the increased use of antiplatelet and antithrombotic medicines, the incidence of acute, subacute, and chronic subdural hematomas is likely to rise in the decades to come. In this issue, leading experts discuss the medical and surgical management of these lesions and provide valuable insights and pearls necessary to achieving the very best outcomes. In addition to reviews on the imaging of these lesions, their epidemiology, and their natural history, this issue provides clinicians with focused articles on complication avoidance and management in a variety of settings, including the outpatient clinic, the ICU, and the operating theater. As there is little class I data on which to base firm recommendations, most discussions will leverage the experience of these highly regarded practitioners and their world-class institutional protocols. The issue ends with an erudite discussion of the issues faced with anticoagulation and how this might be approached when relevant.

E. Sander Connolly Jr, MD
College of Physicians and Surgeons
Columbia University
New York Neurological Institute
NY-Presbyterian Hospital
710 West 168th Street
New York, NY 10032, USA

Guy M. McKhann II, MD
College of Physicians and Surgeons
Columbia University
New York Neurological Institute
NY-Presbyterian Hospital
710 West 168th Street
New York, NY 10032, USA

E-mail addresses:
ESC5@columbia.edu (E.S. Connolly)
GM317@columbia.edu (G.M. McKhann)

Neurosurg Clin N Am 28 (2017) ix
http://dx.doi.org/10.1016/j.nec.2017.01.001
1042-3680/17/© 2017 Published by Elsevier Inc.

Imaging of Subdural Hematomas

Jason J. Carroll, MD[a],*, Sean D. Lavine, MD[b,c], Philip M. Meyers, MD[d]

KEYWORDS

- Imaging • Subdural • Hematoma • CT • MRI

KEY POINTS

- In the early postoperative period, noncontrast head CT is most commonly used to evaluate for potential complications.
- CT is widely available, fast, relatively inexpensive, and accurate at identifying most postoperative complications.
- Intracranial air in the early postoperative period can cause artifact on MRI.
- CT is sensitive for the identification of new intracranial hemorrhage, new mass effect and herniation, tension pneumocephalus, and calvarial fractures.
- Although MRI is less often used in the immediate postoperative period, it is much more sensitive for the detection of acute ischemia and infection.
- The choice to use MRI in the postoperative setting should be driven by the clinical scenario; if acute ischemia or infection is suspected clinically, MRI should always be considered.

BACKGROUND ON IMAGING OF SUBDURAL HEMATOMAS

Historical Imaging Techniques

The imaging of subdural hematoma has evolved significantly. Before modern cross-sectional techniques, such as computed tomography (CT) and MRI, radiography of intracranial pathology generally relied on distortion of normal structures to suggest an intracranial process.[1] Early techniques including plain film radiography, ventriculography, pneumoencephalography, and catheter angiography were limited in the evaluation of the brain parenchyma and surrounding structures given their inherently poor soft tissue resolution. Therefore, the intracranial structures, including the brain parenchyma and ventricles, had the same density on plain film radiography making evaluation for intracranial hemorrhage, tumors, and other intracranial pathologies impossible to visualize. With the exception of plain film radiography, these tests were generally invasive. For example, ventriculography involved drilling a burr hole and directly injecting air into the ventricular system.[2] Pneumoencephalography also relied on similar principles, although the air was instilled into the subarachnoid space of the spine rather than directly into the ventricular system. Both techniques relied on plain film radiography and tomography to evaluate the ventricles to determine ventricular contour irregularities suggesting a mass occupying lesion.[3–5] These studies were uncomfortable for the patient, often inducing vertigo, nausea, and vomiting.

No financial or commercial conflicts of interest for the above listed authors.

[a] Department of Neurological Surgery, Neurological Institute, New York Presbyterian Hospital-Columbia University Medical Center, 710 West 168 Street, New York, NY 10032, USA; [b] Neurointerventional Services, The Valley Hospital Ridgewood, Ridgewood, NJ, USA; [c] Neuroendovascular Services, Department of Neurological Surgery, Neurological Institute, New York Presbyterian Hospital, 710 West 168 Street, New York, NY 10032, USA; [d] Neuroendovascular Services, Department of Neurological Surgery, Neurological Institute, Children's Hospital of New York, New York Presbyterian Hospital, 710 West 168 Street, New York, NY 10032, USA
* Corresponding author.
E-mail address: jjc2272@cumc.columbia.edu

Complication rates were high, and included headache, neck stiffness, meningitis/ventriculitis, altered consciousness, tachycardia, and focal neurologic signs. For these reasons, repeat studies were often not performed given the level of patient discomfort and risks, which limited the evaluation of disease progression over time.[6] Although catheter angiography depicted the cerebral blood vessels with great detail, it too included substantial risks, was plagued by inherently low soft tissue resolution, and also relied on distortion or displacement of the cerebral vasculature to suggest an underlying space-occupying lesion. CT and MRI have supplanted other procedures and rendered most obsolete for the evaluation of intracranial pathology because of ease of use, tremendous soft tissue resolution, safety, and availability.

Current Imaging Recommendations

Noncontrast CT has become the accepted standard of care for the initial evaluation of patient's with suspected subdural hematoma because of widespread availability, rapid acquisition time, and noninvasive nature. Advanced-generation CT scanners now use multiple detectors, helical acquisition, dual-source, and dual-energy techniques, further improving the quality of CT scans while potentially decreasing the radiation dose to patients depending on the type of study performed. MRI generally has a more limited role in the evaluation of acute intracranial hemorrhage, particularly when evaluating subdural hematoma, for practical reasons including availability in most emergency departments. However, MRI offers important features in determining potential secondary causes of subdural hematomas, such as dural-based neoplasms. There is no longer a role for plain film radiography, ventriculography, or pneumoencephalography in the evaluation of traumatic or nontraumatic intracranial hemorrhage.[7]

IMAGING CHARACTERISTICS
General Features

Subdural hematoma is defined as an extra-axial collection of blood products in the subdural space, which is a potential space between the arachnoid and dura mater. The dura mater is the outermost meningeal layer covering the brain parenchyma. The dura is a thin, fibrous covering that extends over the entire brain and is continuous with the periosteum. The dura is reflected along the medial cerebral hemispheres where two layers form the falx cerebri. Similarly, the dura is reflected along the undersurface of the cerebral hemispheres forming the tentorium cerebelli, which divides the supratentorial and infratentorial compartments. The dural venous sinuses travel between the two dural leaflets along the falx cerebri and tentorium cerebelli. Cortical veins draining the brain parenchyma empty into the dural venous sinuses by crossing the subdural space, hence the term bridging veins. Subdural hematomas are usually caused by tearing of these bridging veins.

Trauma is the most common cause of subdural hematoma.[7] Sudden acceleration/deceleration of the head, rapid head rotation, or direct laceration from skull fractures or penetrating projectiles can tear bridging cortical veins. Spontaneous atraumatic subdural hematomas are particularly common in the elderly and people with alcoholism because of the increased incidence of cerebral atrophy in these populations. Cerebral atrophy causes the extra-axial spaces, including the subdural space, to enlarge and the bridging veins to elongate making them more susceptible to injury.[8] Spontaneous subdural hematomas can also occur in patients with coagulopathy and those taking anticoagulant or antithrombotic medications, such as aspirin, clopidogrel, or warfarin.[9] Less common causes of subdural hematoma include dural-based neoplasms, such as meningiomas, hemangiopericytomas, or metastases.[10,11] Intracranial hypotension caused by cerebrospinal fluid (CSF) leak following cranial, spinal, or paranasal sinus surgery is another uncommon cause of atraumatic subdural hematoma.[12,13] Additional rare causes of subdural hematoma include hyponatremic dehydration and dural venous sinus thrombosis.[14–20] In rare circumstances the subdural hematoma is caused by injury to a cortical artery or ruptured vascular lesion, such as an aneurysm or vascular malformation (**Fig. 1**).[21–26] In some circumstances, no clear cause of the subdural hematoma is identified (**Box 1** and **2**).

Anatomic barriers determine the imaging appearance of subdural hematomas. A crescentic extra-axial collection overlying the cerebral convexities is the classic imaging appearance of subdural hematoma. Subdural hematomas often cross calvarial sutures (by contrast with epidural hematomas); however, they rarely cross midline because of continuity of the dural membrane with the falx. Similarly, subdural collections often marginate the falx cerebri medially and tentorium cerebelli inferiorly (**Fig. 2**). Smaller collections of blood can be seen along either the falx cerebri or tentorium cerebelli alone. Without these anatomic barriers, small extra-axial collections overlying the cerebral hemispheres may be difficult to localize accurately into the correct anatomic extra-axial space: epidural, subdural, or subarachnoid. Subdural hematomas tend to distribute diffusely

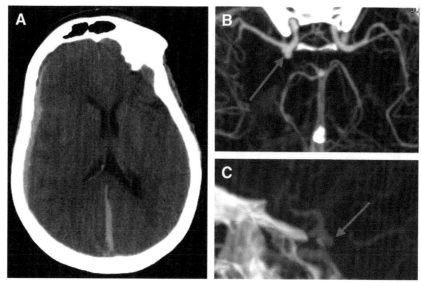

Fig. 1. Noncontrast CT (NCCT) (*A*) demonstrates an acute right convexity subdural hematoma extending along the posterior right falx. Axial (*B*) and sagittal (*C*) maximum intensity projections (MIPs) from a CT angiography demonstrate a bilobed right posterior communicating artery aneurysm (*arrows*) as the cause of the subdural hematoma.

Box 1
Common causes of subdural hematoma

- Trauma
- Spontaneous
  - Elderly (with parenchymal atrophy)
  - Alcoholics (with parenchymal atrophy)
  - Coagulopathic (underlying clotting disorder, liver failure, and so forth)
  - Coagulopathic caused by blood thinning medications
- Idiopathic

throughout the potential space between the dura and arachnoid meningeal layers. By contrast, adherence of the dura to the periosteum limits the spread of blood products, giving epidural collections their more focal and biconvex shape. This anatomy also explains why epidural collections do not cross suture lines because the dura mater is densely adherent to the inner table of the

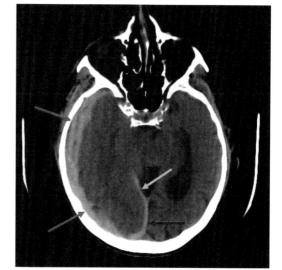

Fig. 2. NCCT demonstrates a heterogeneously hyperdense acute right convexity subdural hematoma (*red arrows*) extending along the right posterior falx (*blue arrow*) and posterior right tentorial leaflet (*green arrow*).

Box 2
Rare causes of subdural hematomas

Dural-based neoplasms (eg, meningioma, hemangiopericytoma, metastasis)

Intracranial hypotension

Hyponatremic dehydration

Vascular lesions (eg, aneurysm, dural arteriovenous fistula, arteriovenous malformation)

Dural venous sinus thrombosis

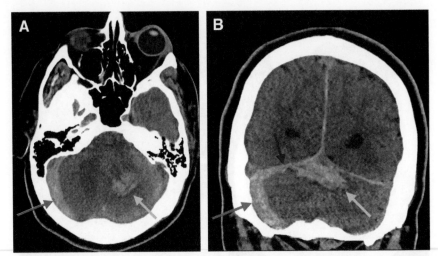

Fig. 3. Axial (*A*) and coronal (*B*) NCCT demonstrates an acute subdural hematoma along the right cerebellar convexity (*red arrows*) extending along the inferior right tentorial leaflet (*blue arrow*). Also note the acute parenchymal hematoma in the paramedian cerebellum (*green arrows*).

calvarium at the sutures. Exceptions to these imaging guidelines may be seen with dural hypoplasia or trauma. Subarachnoid hemorrhage is distinguishable from subdural hematomas by its extension within the subarachnoid spaces, and characteristic presence in cerebral cisterns and sulci. Subdural hematomas can also occur, albeit less frequently, in the posterior fossa and spinal canal. Posterior fossa subdural hematomas have a similar imaging appearance to supratentorial subdural collections (**Fig. 3**). Subdural hematomas can sometimes be seen in the upper cervical spine on the caudal-most slices of a head CT or MRI. Therefore, careful evaluation of the upper cervical

spine at the margin of cross-sectional imaging must be performed to identify spinal lesions.

Computed Tomography Characteristics

The appearance of blood products on CT changes according to their radiodensity as measured in Hounsfield units (HU). This density depends predominantly on the age of the hemorrhage and stage of blood degradation. Therefore, most subdural hematomas follow a fairly predictable course on serial CT scanning. Most acute subdural hematomas are hyperdense compared with the cerebral cortex (**Fig. 4**). The density decreases by

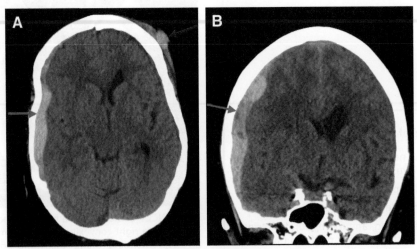

Fig. 4. Axial (*A*) and coronal (*B*) NCCT of traumatic acute right convexity subdural hematoma (*red arrows*). Notice the left frontal subgaleal hematoma (*blue arrow*) indicating the contrecoup nature of the subdural hematoma.

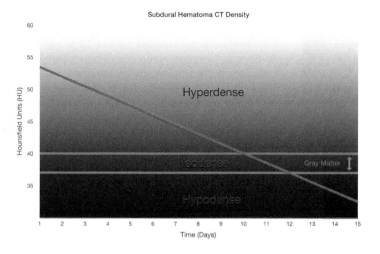

Fig. 5. Subdural hematoma CT density.

Table 1
CT density of common substances measured in Hounsfield units

Substance	CT Density (HU)
Air	−1000 to −600
Fat	−100 to −60
Water	0
CSF	15
Kidney	30
Muscle	10–40
White matter	20–30
Gray matter	37–45
Acute blood	50–80
Liver	40–60
Bone	>700

approximately 1.5 HU per day (**Fig. 5**, **Table 1**). Therefore, by Days 7 to 10, the hematoma are approximately isodense to the cerebral cortex (**Fig. 6**), and by Days 10 to 14 should be hypodense relative to cortex (**Fig. 7**).[27,28] Several confounding factors can affect the apparent density of subdural hematomas on CT making age determination inaccurate.[7] These factors include hyperacute blood (active bleeding), coagulopathy preventing clotting, CSF leakage through torn arachnoid membranes that dilutes blood and limits dense clot formation, blood products of varying ages, profound anemia, and superimposed infection (**Box 3**).

MRI Characteristics

Age determination and signal characteristics of subdural hematomas on MRI are more complex

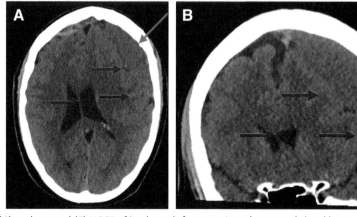

Fig. 6. Axial (*A*) and coronal (*B*) NCCT of isodense left convexity subacute subdural hematoma (*red arrows*). Notice the sulcal and ventricular effacement deep to the subdural collection (*blue arrows*).

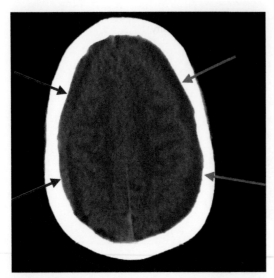

Fig. 7. NCCT of hypodense left convexity chronic subdural hematoma (*red arrows*). Also notice the subacute right convexity subdural hematoma with subtle hematocrit gradation (*blue arrows*).

and less predictable than CT density. The variable MRI appearance of subdural hematoma is related to hemoglobin structure and its oxidation products. Hemoglobin passes through various forms during red blood cell lysis including intracellular oxyhemoglobin, intracellular deoxyhemoglobin, intracellular methemoglobin, extracellular methemoglobin, and finally extracellular ferritin and hemosiderin. These forms roughly correlate with blood products in the hyperacute (<24 hours), acute (24–72 hours), early subacute (3–7 days), late subacute (7–14 days), and chronic stages (>14 days), respectively (**Fig. 8**). However, accurate dating of subdural hematoma is sometimes difficult and inaccurate because of heterogeneity of the oxidation progression.[29–32]

Multiple forms of hemoglobin are often found in a single hematoma. The paramagnetic dipole-dipole interactions of methemoglobin are

Box 3
Confounding factors in aging of subdural hematoma on CT
Unclotted, active bleeding (often in patients with coagulopathy)
CSF leakage
Anemia
Blood products of varying ages
Superimposed infection

responsible for the T1 hyperintense signal seen in the subacute phase, whereas magnetic susceptibility effect is responsible for the T2 signal loss (hypointensity) seen in the acute (deoxyhemoglobin), early subacute (intracellular methemoglobin), and chronic (hemosiderin) stages of blood product evolution. Additionally, as the protein content of the hematoma increases over time, so does the T2 hypointensity (see **Fig. 8**). Subdural hematomas are often hyperintense in the acute, subacute, and chronic stages on fluid attenuated inversion recovery (FLAIR) images, whereas the signal characteristics are variable in the hyperacute stage. Hematomas are usually hypointense on gradient echo (GRE), T2*, and susceptibility-weighted images (SWI) caused by magnetic susceptibility effects. GRE, T2*, and susceptibility sequences are exquisitely sensitive for the detection of chronic blood products. The magnetic susceptibility effects are enhanced with higher field strength magnets (3T and 7T), whereas fast spin echo techniques dampen the effects. Subdural hematomas in all stages often contain various amounts of hyperintense signal on diffusion weighted (DWI) images, which is often caused by magnetic susceptibility artifact. DWI hyperintensity should not be confused with superimposed infection, unless clinical circumstances warrants such consideration.[29–32]

ACUTE SUBDURAL HEMATOMA
Overview of Imaging Characteristics by Time (Days 0–3)

An acute subdural hematoma is defined as being zero to approximately several days old. Acute subdural hematomas are one of the leading causes of morbidity and mortality in patients with severe traumatic brain injury.[7] Traumatic acute subdural hematomas are often accompanied by other types of intracranial hemorrhage, such as subarachnoid hemorrhage, intraventricular hemorrhage, parenchymal contusions, and epidural hematomas.

Noncontrast Head Computed Tomography Findings

Most (60%) acute subdural hematomas are hyperdense relative to gray matter with Hounsfield units typically ranging from 50 to 80.[7] It is helpful to use "wide" (subdural) windowing (window, 175; level, 50) and "narrow" (brain) windowing (window, 80; level, 40) to separate hyperdense blood products from adjacent cortex (**Fig. 9**). Up to 40% of acute subdural hematomas have a mixed hyperdense and hypodense appearance (**Fig. 10**). The hypodensity may reflect unclotted blood products, CSF leakage through torn arachnoid membranes,

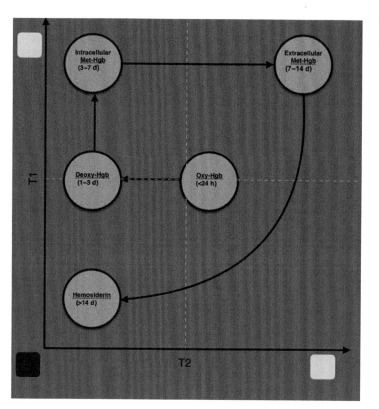

Fig. 8. MRI signal characteristics of aging subdural hematoma.

or profound anemia.[33] A "swirl sign," which appears as irregular pockets of hypodensity within the dominant hyperdense collection, is most often associated with rapid, active bleeding (**Fig. 11**).[34]

In patients with coagulopathy or anemia, the collections may rarely be isodense with respect to underlying brain parenchyma making detection more challenging.[35,36]

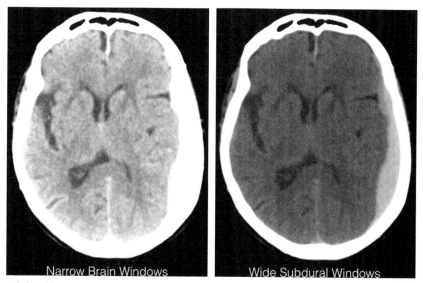

Fig. 9. Acute subdural hematoma in narrow brain (window, 175; level, 50) and wide subdural (window, 80; level, 40) windows. Notice how the hyperdense subdural hematoma is indistinguishable from the calvarium with the narrow brain window.

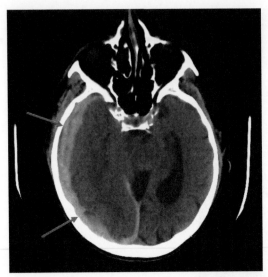

Fig. 10. NCCT demonstrates a predominantly hyperdense acute right convexity subdural hematoma with scattered areas of hypodensity (*red arrows*).

MRI Findings

Acute subdural hematomas are often T1 isointense and T2 hypointense because of intracellular deoxyhemoglobin. If MRI is performed less than 24 hours after hematoma formation, the collection may be T1 isointense and T2 hyperintense because of intracellular oxyhemoglobin. Acute subdural hematomas on T2-weighted FLAIR images are usually isointense-to-hypointense relative to normal CSF. Therefore, FLAIR sequences are not as sensitive as CT to identify acute subdural hematoma because small collections may be indistinguishable from normal adjacent CSF. GRE and susceptibility sequences often show at least a rim of "blooming" hypointensity. DWI is often hyperintense, whereas the ADC map is highly variable (**Fig. 12**).[29–31]

Computed Tomography/Magnetic Resonance Angiography Findings

Although CT angiography (CTA) and magnetic resonance angiography (MRA) are not frequently performed in the setting of an isolated acute subdural hematoma, they may be indicated in the setting of trauma to evaluate for vascular injury (arterial or venous), particularly when calvarial and skull base fractures course through vascular foramen (eg, carotid canal) or dural venous sinuses. When calvarial fractures traverse dural venous sinuses, particularly occipital fractures involving the transverse sinuses, it may be difficult to distinguish between small epidural and subdural hematomas. In these cases, CTA and less commonly MRA can be helpful to localize the extra-axial collection: epidural hematomas displace the cortical veins and dural venous sinuses inward, whereas subdural hematoma displaces the dural venous sinus outward toward the calvarium (**Figs. 13 and 14**). CTA may also demonstrate an angiographic "spot sign," which

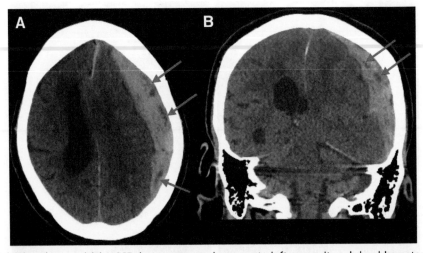

Fig. 11. Axial (*A*) and coronal (*B*) NCCT demonstrates a large acute left convexity subdural hematoma with evidence of a "swirl" sign concerning for rapid, active extravasation. Scattered pockets of hypodensity within the predominantly hyperdense subdural hematoma are consistent with unclotted blood (*arrows*). Note the pronounced midline shift and right lateral ventricular trapping.

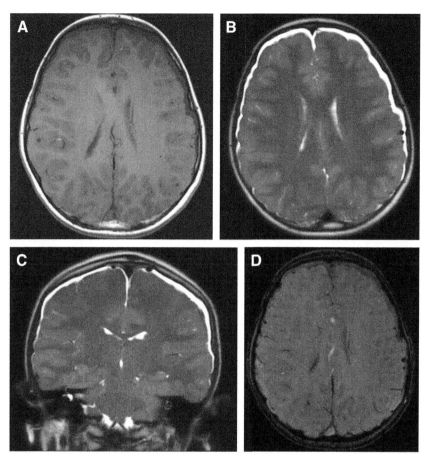

Fig. 12. MRI in a 7-year-old trauma patient demonstrates bilateral acute subdural hematomas that are T1 isointense (*A*) and T2 hyperintense (*B, C*) to cortex with scattered blooming on susceptibility-weighted images (*D*).

indicates active extravasation from a cortical vessel. The angiographic "spot sign" is more commonly associated with active extravasation in acute parenchymal hematomas.[37]

SUBACUTE SUBDURAL HEMATOMAS
Overview of Imaging Characteristics by Time (Days 3–14)

A subacute subdural hematoma is defined as being approximately 3 to 14 days old. The collection has a similar distribution as an acute subdural hematoma, often crescentic in shape overlying a cerebral hemisphere with or without extension along the falx and tentorium. The once soft, loosely organized clot begins to organize as hemoglobin degradation begins. Neomembranes of granulation tissue begin to form along the periphery of the clot. Repetitive hemorrhage at this stage may be related to bridging cortical venous bleeding, whether new or recurrent, or from the friable neomembranes that are becoming adherent to the dura and arachnoid.

Noncontrast Head Computed Tomography Findings

As the hematoma organizes and protein degradation occurs the collection becomes progressively hypodense on CT. Eventually (usually 10–14 days), in the absence of new hemorrhage, the hematoma becomes isodense with the adjacent cortex (**Figs. 15** and **16**). At this stage the collection is indistinguishable in density from gray matter on CT, particularly if small in size or bilateral in nature, which can produce opposing mass effect preventing midline shift. Subtle signs of balanced mass effect, such as sulcal effacement or slitlike ventricles, may be the only clues as to the presence of bilateral subacute subdural collections. Subacute subdural hematomas are often mixed attenuation because of blood products in various stages of evolution, making them easier to identify (**Fig. 17**).[28] Subtle hematocrit gradation within the hematoma is common at this stage with more hyperdense blood products seen layering dependently (see **Fig. 7**).

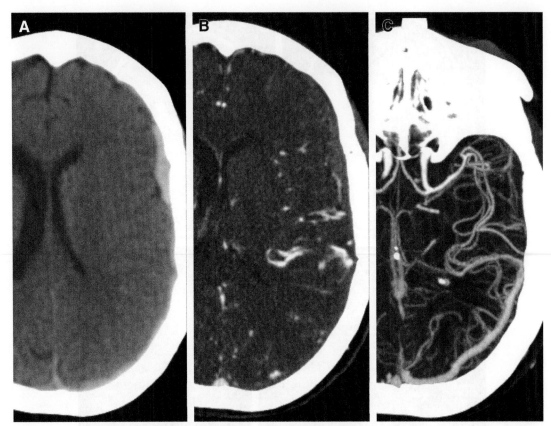

Fig. 13. Acute left convexity subdural hematoma on NCCT (*A*), CTA source images (*B*), and CTA MIP images (*C*). Notice how the cortical veins on the left are displaced medially away from the calvarium.

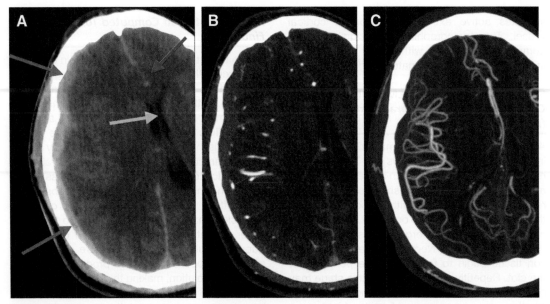

Fig. 14. NCCT (*A*), CTA source images (*B*), and CTA MIP images (*C*) demonstrate an acute right convexity subdural hematoma (*red arrows*). Notice the medial displacement of the cortical vessels (*blue arrows*), significant midline shift (*green arrow*), and subfalcine herniation (*pink arrow*).

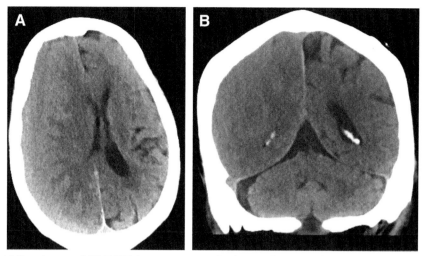

Fig. 15. Axial (*A*) and coronal (*B*) NCCT demonstrates an isodense subacute right convexity subdural hematoma. Note the obliteration of sulci in the right cerebral hemisphere, effacement of the right lateral ventricle, and leftward midline shift.

MRI Findings

Early subacute subdural hematomas (approximately Days 3–7) are often T1 isointense-to-hyperintense and T2 hypointense to cortex because of intracellular methemoglobin being the predominant hemoglobin breakdown product present at this stage (**Fig. 18**). The hematoma gradually becomes more T1 and T2 hyperintense as extracellular methemoglobin predominates (**Figs. 19** and **20**). T2-weighted FLAIR images are exquisitely sensitive at identifying even the smallest of subacute subdural hematomas because the collections are very hyperintense. GRE and SWI demonstrates marked "blooming." Early subacute subdural hematomas are often hyperintense on DWI, whereas later subacute subdural hematomas are not. Contrast-enhanced T1-weighted images may show smooth, linear enhancement along the margins of the subdural collection corresponding to developing granulation tissue and neomembranes (**Fig. 21**). Smooth, thin enhancement should not be confused with superimposed subdural empyema except in the appropriate clinical setting. MRI during this stage of clot evolution is helpful in identifying subdural collections that

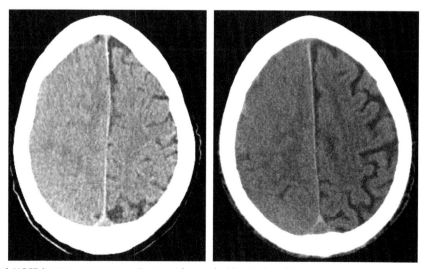

Fig. 16. Axial NCCT in two separate patients with nearly identical right convexity isodense subacute subdural hematomas.

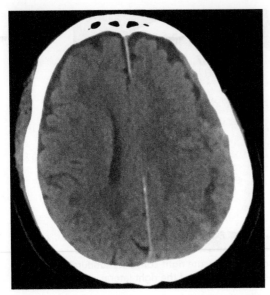

Fig. 17. NCCT demonstrates a mixed density subacute left convexity subdural hematoma.

are isodense on CT, particularly if bilateral (**Fig. 22**).[29–31]

CHRONIC SUBDURAL HEMATOMAS/ HYGROMAS
Overview of Imaging Characteristics by Time (Days 15–21)

Chronic subdural hematomas are defined as being greater than 2 to 3 weeks old. As the hematoma continues to evolve and blood products degrade, the collection becomes increasingly liquefied with accumulation of sanguineous or serosanguineous fluid centrally along with progressive maturation of a thick, fibrous capsule. Therefore, the collection becomes increasingly CSF-like on imaging. Repeat hemorrhage caused by stretching and tearing of the bridging cortical veins or encapsulated membranes is common, often giving the collection a mixed appearance on CT and MRI. Mixed-attenuation subdural collections on CT, known as "acute-on-chronic" subdural hematomas, are discussed in detail in the next section.

In contrast to subdural hematoma, a subdural hygroma is a collection of CSF in the subdural space resulting from traumatic arachnoid tearing or passive effusion in the setting of spontaneous intracranial hypotension, dehydration, or brain parenchymal atrophy. Subdural hygromas are indistinguishable from chronic subdural hematomas on CT because both appear homogeneously hypodense. The subdural collections are distinguished on MRI because chronic subdural

hematomas show evidence of chronic blood products, whereas subdural hygromas follow CSF on all pulse-sequences (**Figs. 23** and **24**). Subdural hygromas may become large enough and produce enough mass effect to warrant surgical drainage.

Chronic subdural hematomas or subdural hygromas can potentially be difficult to distinguish from prominence of the extra-axial spaces because of brain parenchymal atrophy. The lack of mass effect, including cortical buckling and sulcal effacement, may not always exclude a subdural collection because patients with substantial parenchymal atrophy can accommodate large amounts of subdural hemorrhage or CSF without significant mass effect. One particularly useful clue that favors brain parenchymal volume loss over a subdural collection is the presence of cortical vessels traversing the hypodensity, which would be displaced if a subdural collection is present. One must be careful not to mistake septations associated with chronic subdural hematomas for cortical vessels.[28,38]

Noncontrast Head Computed Tomography Findings

A chronic subdural hematoma without evidence of recurrent hemorrhage appears as a nearly homogeneous, hypodense subdural collection with or without gravity-dependent hematocrit gradation (see **Fig. 7**; **Fig. 25**).[39] These types of chronic subdural hematomas may be indistinguishable from subdural hygromas on CT alone. Prior imaging can be instrumental in drawing the distinction between these two. If prior imaging clearly demonstrates blood products in the subdural space, then the hypodense subdural collection is a chronic subdural hematoma.[6,27]

Some chronic subdural hematomas demonstrate internal septations and appear loculated. The thick internal septations and capsule appear hyperdense on CT (see **Fig. 25**). The hyperdensity should not be confused with recurrent hemorrhage. Long-standing chronic subdural hematomas may appear as diffuse hyperdense dural thickening caused by near complete resorption of the liquefied blood products centrally. The "thickened dura" can become coarsely calcified over time (**Fig. 26**).[7,28]

MRI Findings

Continued oxidative denaturation of methemoglobin forms nonparamagnetic hemichromes, also known as "hemoglobin breakdown products." The T1 signal of such breakdown products is less pronounced than methemoglobin, leading

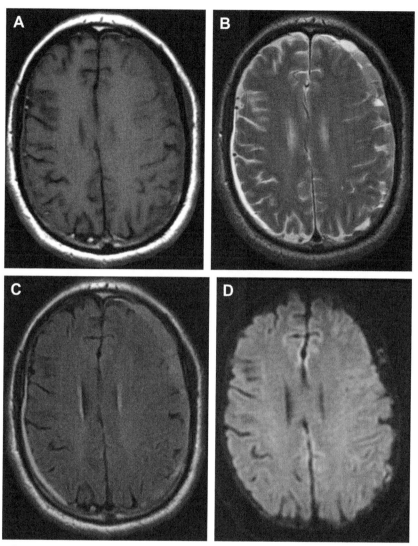

Fig. 18. Early subacute left convexity subdural hematoma that is isointense to cortex with scattered hyperintensity on T1-weighted image (*A*), predominantly isointense on T2-weighted image (*B*), and mildly hyperintense on FLAIR images (*C*) with scattered DWI hyperintense signal (*D*).

to progressively hypointense T1 signal. The T1 signal is always greater than CSF because of higher protein content of the subdural collection. The T2 signal also becomes progressively hypointense because of the combination of magnetic susceptibility effect and elevated protein. The collection eventually becomes isointense-to-hypointense relative to CSF on T2-weighted images. A rim of hemosiderin develops less frequently in subdural hematomas compared with parenchymal hematomas because tissue macrophages, which are responsible for the storage of iron as ferritin or hemosiderin, are not sequestered in the extra-axial spaces.

Approximately one-quarter of chronic subdural hematomas develop superficial siderosis on GRE and SWI.[29] Most chronic subdural hematomas remain hyperintense on T2-weighted FLAIR images. No DWI restriction should be seen in uncomplicated chronic subdural hematomas. The presence of DWI restriction could indicate repeat hemorrhage, subacute blood products, or superimposed infection. The fibrous capsule and internal septations enhance avidly on postcontrast T1-weighted images. As previously mentioned, subdural hygromas should follow CSF on all pulse sequences without evidence of blood products, particularly on GRE or SWI.[30,31,38,40]

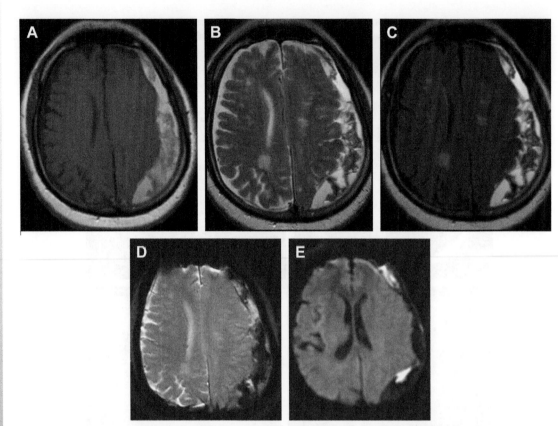

Fig. 19. Late subacute left convexity subdural hematoma with predominantly extracellular methemoglobin this is hyperintense in T1-weighted (*A*), mixed hyperintense and hypointense on T2-weighted and FLAIR images (*B, C*), and demonstrates blooming susceptibility artifact on gradient echo images (*D*). Heterogeneous DWI hyperintense signal is caused by susceptibility artifact (*E*). Note the internal septations that are beginning to form.

MIXED/ACUTE-ON-CHRONIC SUBDURAL HEMATOMAS
Overview of Imaging Characteristics

Most subdural hematomas do not demonstrate perfectly homogeneous attenuation on CT or MRI. Some heterogeneity is attributed to hemoglobin degradation not uniform throughout the collection. Therefore, the imaging characteristics and timeline of acute, subacute, and chronic subdural hematomas on CT and MRI previously described are rough guidelines. Recurrent hemorrhage into an existing subdural hematoma accounts for additional heterogeneity within a subdural collection. Not infrequently, blood products in the acute, subacute, and chronic stages are seen within a single subdural collection.[41,42]

Acute rehemorrhage into an existing chronic subdural hematoma, known simply as an acute-on-chronic subdural hematoma, may result from new tearing of bridging cortical veins or bleeding from friable membranes encapsulating a chronic subdural hematoma. Hyperacute active hemorrhage, coagulopathy, superimposed infection, and CSF leakage into a subdural hematoma can also lead to mixed attenuation.

Computed Tomography Findings

The most common appearance of an acute-on-chronic subdural hematoma is a crescentic subdural collection overlying a cerebral hemisphere with distinct gravity-dependent hematocrit level known as a "hematocrit effect" (**Figs. 27** and **28**). Hyperdense acute blood products layer dependently, whereas more chronic blood products are seen antidependently.[43,44]

The acute-on-chronic appearance is different from gravity-dependent hematocrit gradient seen in subacute subdural hematomas. Acute-on-chronic subdural hematomas may also show more scattered areas of acute hyperdense blood products within a hypodense chronic subdural collection (**Figs. 29–31**). Compartmentalized

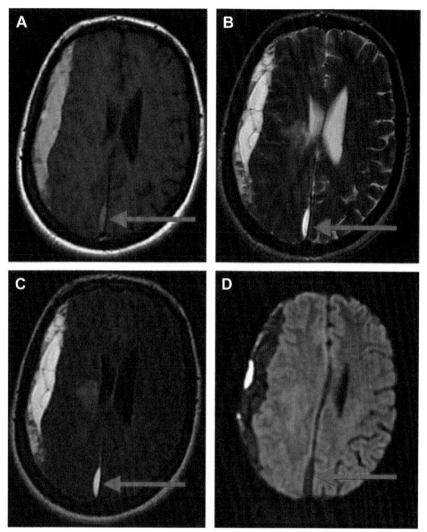

Fig. 20. Late subacute right convexity subdural hematoma with internal septations and multiloculated appearance. The collection is hyperintense on T1 (*A*), T2 (*B*), and FLAIR (*C*) sequences, although it is predominantly hypointense with scattered areas of hyperintensity on DWI (*D*). Note the extension along the right posterior falx (*arrows*).

pockets of acute blood products in multiloculated chronic subdural collections can sometimes create the appearance of loculated collections with fluid-fluid levels and irregular internal septations (**Fig. 32**).[39]

MRI Findings

The MRI appearance of mixed subdural hematomas is highly variable, depending on the hemoglobin breakdown stage of the new blood products and degree of organization. Acute-on-chronic subdural hematomas may have a hematocrit level similar to that seen on CT, and can also appear heterogeneous, if multiloculated compartments and blood products in various stage of

evolution are present. The T1 and T2 characteristics are highly dependent on the stage of hemoglobin degradation among other factors. Blooming is often seen on GRE and SWI. T2-weighted FLAIR images are often hyperintense. Restricted diffusion is common on DWI because acute or subacute blood products are usually present. The fibrous capsule and internal septations enhance avidly on postcontrast T1-weighted images (**Table 2**).[31,40]

IMAGING OF SECONDARY EFFECTS OF SUBDURAL HEMATOMA

Identifying and accurately characterizing intracranial hemorrhage, including subdural hematomas,

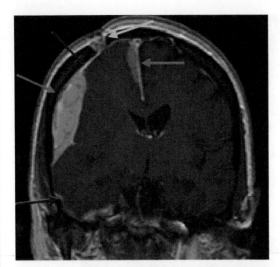

Fig. 21. Coronal T1 postcontrast image demonstrates an intrinsically T1 hyperintense late subacute right convexity subdural hematoma extending along the right falx (*red arrows*). Note the smooth, thin dural enhancement over the right cerebral convexity (*blue arrows*). Also note the right frontal burr hole related to prior hematoma evacuation (*green arrow*).

are the first steps but not the only imaging considerations when evaluating patients with intracranial hemorrhage. The secondary effects are the reason subdural hematomas can become life-threatening, and features apparent on imaging studies often guide medical and surgical management. Secondary effects are primarily related to mass effect on the intracranial structures.

Initially, subdural hematomas displace and compress the underlying brain parenchyma, cerebral sulci, and ventricles. The earliest signs of mass effect include cortical "buckling" and sulcal and ventricular effacement with or without midline shift. As mass effect progresses, midline shift begins to occur without associated herniation. An accurate measurement of midline shift is critical to clinical management and should always be documented.[43] The best way to determine the native midline is to draw a straight line between the anterior and posterior attachments of the falx cerebri with the inner table of the calvarium along the frontal and occipital crests. A separate perpendicular line can then be drawn from the native midline to the displaced midline structures. The septum

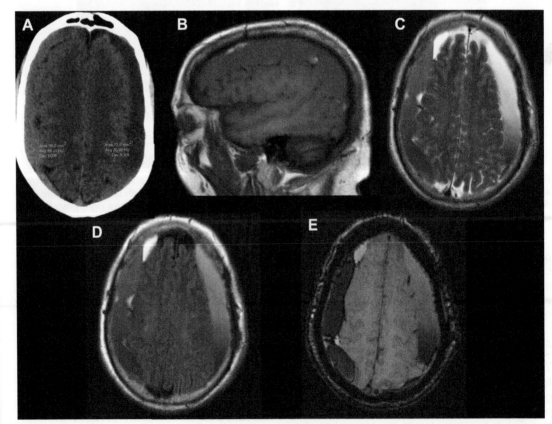

Fig. 22. NCCT (*A*) and MRI demonstrate early subacute right convexity and late subacute left convexity subdural hematomas. Note the scattered hyperintense methemoglobin on T1-weighted image (*B*), intracellular methemoglobin in the right convexity collection and extracellular methemoglobin in the left convexity collection on T2-weighted image (*C*), heterogeneous appearance on FLAIR images (*D*), and right greater than left blooming on susceptibility-weighted images (*E*).

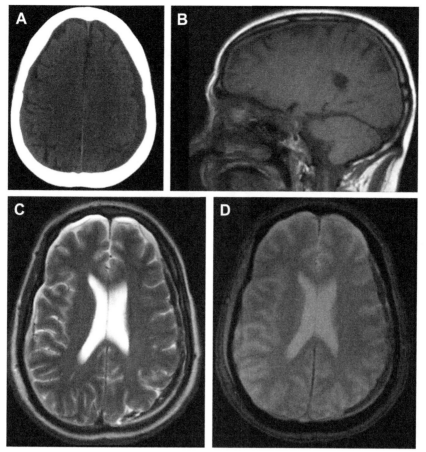

Fig. 23. NCCT (*A*) and multisequence MRI demonstrates a T1 isointense (*B*) and T2 hypointense (*C*) to cortex chronic left convexity subdural hematoma with slight blooming on gradient echo images (*D*).

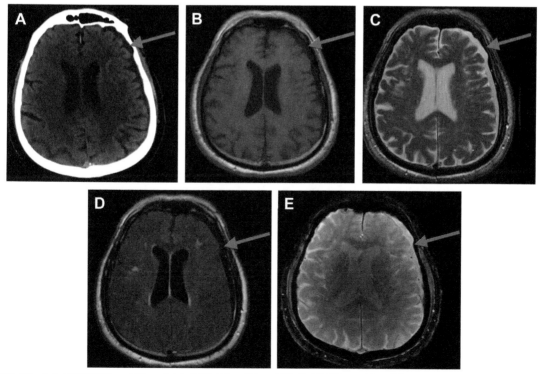

Fig. 24. Axial NCCT (*A*) and T1-weighted (*B*), T2-weighted (*C*), FLAIR (*D*), and SWI (*E*) MRI sequences demonstrate a small left convexity subdural hygroma (*arrows*) that follows CSF on all MRI pulse sequences.

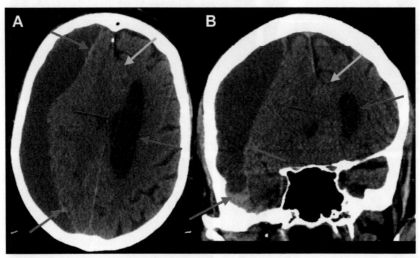

Fig. 25. Axial (*A*) and coronal (*B*) NCCT demonstrate a large chronic hypodense right convexity subdural hematoma. Notice the thin capsule that appears slightly hyperdense in certain areas (*red arrows*). Also note the significant midline shift (*blue arrows*), subfalcine herniation (*green arrows*), and left lateral ventricular trapping resulting in hydrocephalus (*pink arrows*).

pellucidum between the lateral ventricles is often the easiest estimate of the displaced midline, although other surrogates, such as the displaced interhemispheric fissure, can also be used (**Fig. 33**). As mass effect becomes increasingly severe, various herniation syndromes and their sequelae develop.

Herniation Syndromes

The most common herniation syndromes include subfalcine, descending and ascending transtentorial, and tonsillar. Less common herniation syndromes include transalar and transcranial. The focus here is on the more common herniation syndromes: subfalcine, transtentorial, and tonsillar.

Subfalcine herniation
Subfalcine herniation is the most common herniation syndrome. It occurs when a space-occupying lesion in the supratentorial compartment exerts transverse mass effect such that the brain parenchyma and accompanying cerebral blood vessels

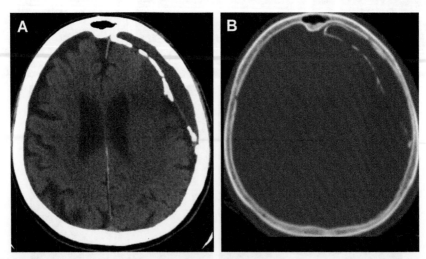

Fig. 26. Axial NCCT in subdural (*A*) and bone (*B*) windows demonstrates a peripherally calcified chronic left frontal convexity subdural hematoma.

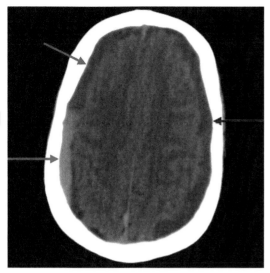

Fig. 27. NCCT demonstrates an acute-on-chronic right convexity subdural hematoma with hematocrit effect (*red arrows*) and chronic left convexity subdural hematoma (*blue arrow*).

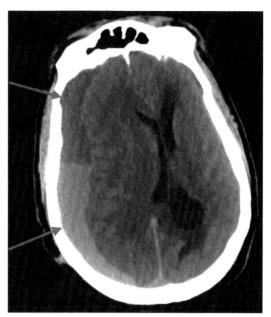

Fig. 28. NCCT demonstrates an acute-on-chronic right convexity subdural hematoma with hematocrit effect (*arrows*).

herniate below the free edge of the falx cerebri into the contralateral supratentorial compartment. Subdural hematomas are a common cause of subfalcine herniation (see **Figs. 11, 14, 25, 28, 30; Fig. 34**).

The paired anterior cerebral arteries (ACAs) coursing in the interhemispheric fissure are usually displaced with herniated brain parenchyma. In severe cases, the ACA (one or both) may be compressed against the rigid free edge of the falx cerebri, which may lead to an ACA territory infarction. Therefore, close evaluation of the brain parenchyma in the ACA territories in cases of subfalcine herniation is critical in early identification of ACA territory infarctions.

As the subfalcine herniation progresses, so does the effacement and compression of the lateral ventricles. Eventually, the mass effects occludes the contralateral foramen of Monro resulting in contralateral obstructive hydrocephalus. This often manifests as asymmetric dilatation of the frontal horn of the contralateral lateral ventricle,

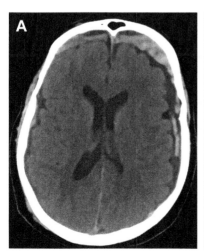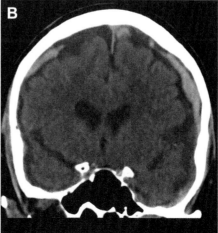

Fig. 29. Axial (*A*) and coronal (*B*) NCCT demonstrate bilateral acute-on-chronic subdural hematomas.

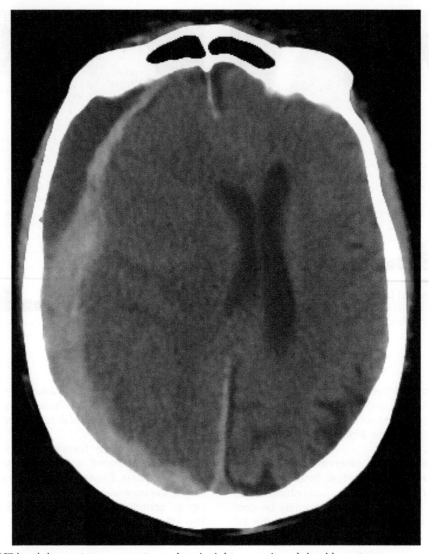

Fig. 30. NCCT head demonstrates an acute-on-chronic right convexity subdural hematoma.

although involvement of the atrium and temporal horn can also occur depending on the site of ventricular obstruction (see **Figs. 2, 4, 10, 11, 25, 28, 32,** and **34**).[7,39,45]

Descending transtentorial herniation

Descending transtentorial herniation occurs when a space-occupying supratentorial lesion exerts enough medial and downward pressure on the medial temporal lobe to displace it over the free edge of the ipsilateral tentorial leaflet through the tentorial incisura. Medial displacement of the temporal lobe initially effaces the ipsilateral ambient (perimesencephalic) and suprasellar cisterns, and eventually leads to effacement of the quadrigeminal cistern as the

herniation progresses (see **Fig. 10** and **34**). In severe cases, brainstem compression results in obtundation, diminished respiratory drive, cranial neuropathies, and ultimately death. Severe mass effect may also result in bilateral descending transtentorial herniation as manifested by bilateral brainstem compression and complete effacement of the basilar cisterns on imaging (**Fig. 35**).

The P2 and P3 segments of the posterior cerebral arteries (PCA) traverse the midbrain via the ambient and quadrigeminal cisterns. In doing so, the PCAs are susceptible to compression and possible infarction as the medial temporal lobes herniate over the free edge of the tentorial leaflets. Therefore, close evaluation of the brain

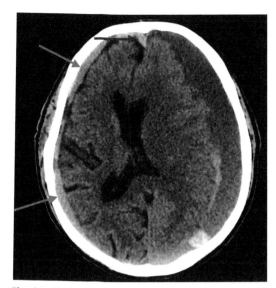

Fig. 31. NCCT demonstrates an acute-on-chronic left convexity subdural hematoma. Also note the acute right convexity subdural hematoma (*red arrows*) extending along the right anterior falx (*blue arrow*).

temporal lobe, which may cause ipsilateral hemiparesis. Indentation of the contralateral cereberal peduncle in such cases is known as Kernohan notch (see **Fig. 34**).

Pressure effects secondary to severe descending transtentorial herniation can cause pressure necrosis of the uncus and hippocampus; hypothalamic and basal ganglia infarcts caused by compression of perforating arteries arising from the proximal circle of Willis; and hemorrhagic infarction of the ventral pons and midbrain, which results from compression and occlusion of basilar perforating arteries along the ventral pons and midbrain, often called Duret hemorrhages.[7,39,45]

Ascending transtentorial herniation

Ascending transtentorial herniation is less common and occurs when a space-occupying lesion in the posterior fossa causes upward displacement of the cerebellar vermis and medial cerebellar hemispheres superiorly through the tentorial incisura. The midbrain is displaced ventrally, and the mass effect results in effacement of the quadrigeminal cistern, fourth ventricle, and cerebral aqueduct causing obstructive hydrocephalus (see **Fig. 35**). Posterior fossa tumors and swelling associated with ischemic cerebellar infarcts are the most common causes of upward transtentorial herniation. Posterior fossa hemorrhage, particularly parenchymal hematomas, can cause upward transtentorial herniation. However, posterior fossa subdural hematomas are a rare cause of upward transtentorial herniation (see **Fig. 3**; **Fig. 36**).[39,46]

parenchyma in the PCA territory ipsilateral to the descending transtentorial herniation is crucial in identifying early signs of cerebral infarction. Angiography, both catheter and noninvasive (CTA or MRA), may show inferior displacement, narrowing, and possible occlusion of the affected PCA.

Severe descending transtentorial herniation can eventually cause compression of the contralateral cerebral peduncle against the contralateral medial

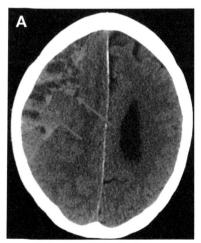
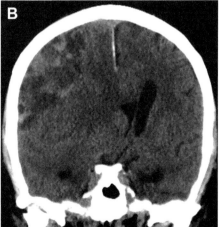

Fig. 32. Axial (*A*) and coronal (*B*) NCCT demonstrates a multiloculated acute-on-chronic right frontal convexity subdural hematoma. Note the compartmentalized hyperdense acute blood products layering dependently (*arrows*).

Table 2
MRI and CT characteristics of subdural hematomas

Subdural Hematomas Age	Hemoglobin Form	CT Density	T1	T2
Hyperacute (<24 h)	Oxyhemoglobin	Hyperdense	Isodense to hypointense	Hyperintense
Acute (24–72 h)	Deoxyhemoglobin	Hyperdense	Isodense to hypointense	Hypointense
Early subacute (3–7 d)	Methemoglobin (intracellular)	Hyperdense to isodense	Hyperintense	Hypointense
Late subacute (7–14 d)	Methemoglobin (extracellular)	Isodense to hypodense	Hyperintense	Hyperintense
Chronic (>14 d)	Ferritin and hemosiderin	Hypodense	Hypointense	Hypointense

Acquired tonsillar herniation

Acquired tonsillar herniation occurs when a posterior fossa space-occupying lesion results in caudal herniation of the cerebellar tonsils through the foramen magnum. This may occur simultaneously with ascending transtentorial herniation and from similar causes, such as posterior fossa tumors and swelling related to ischemic cerebellar infarcts. Posterior fossa hemorrhage, particularly subdural hematomas, are less common causes of acquired tonsillar herniation. Sagittal cross-sectional images, whether CT or MRI, best demonstrate tonsillar herniation, although axial imaging nicely demonstrates the cerebellar tonsils completely filling the foramen magnum in cases of tonsillar herniation (see **Fig. 36**).[7,39,45]

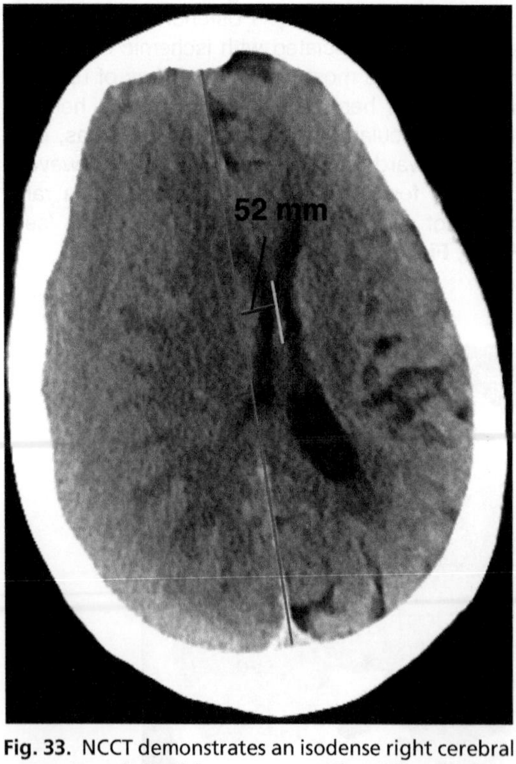

Fig. 33. NCCT demonstrates an isodense right cerebral convexity subdural hematoma with midline shift as measured with a perpendicular line (*blue line*) drawn from the native midline (*red line*) to the displaced midline represented by the septum pellucidum (*green line*).

52 mm

Obstructive hydrocephalus

Obstructive hydrocephalus caused by herniation syndromes is a life-threatening sequela of subdural hematomas. Lateral ventricular obstructive hydrocephalus caused by substantial midline shift resulting in ventricular trapping is the most common pattern of hydrocephalus associated with large supratentorial subdural hematomas (see **Figs. 2**, **4**, **10**, **11**, **25**, **28**, **32**, and **34**). The entire contralateral lateral ventricle may be dilated, but more often focal dilatation of the frontal or temporal horns occurs depending on the site of trapping. Cerebral infarction may eventually result. Enlargement of the temporal horns of the lateral ventricles is one of the first clues in identifying early obstructive hydrocephalus. The temporal horns are subtle or not visualized in normal, young patients because of normal brain parenchymal volume. In elderly patients and those with underlying conditions causing parenchymal atrophy, recognition of early hydrocephalus may be challenging and overdiagnosis of hydrocephalus may occur because of prominence of the ventricular system secondary to central atrophy. Comparison with a prior studies, if available, is always helpful to evaluate for changes in ventricular size.[7,39,45]

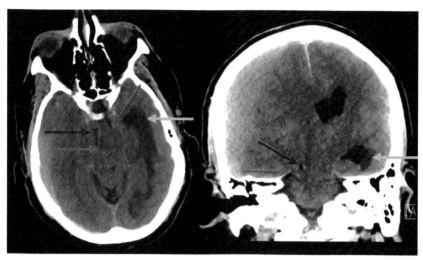

Fig. 34. Axial (*A*) and coronal (*B*) NCCT demonstrates a large acute-on-chronic right convexity subdural hematoma resulting in marked midline shift and right descending transtentorial herniation (*red arrows*) with complete effacement of the basilar cisterns, midbrain compression, and obstructive hydrocephalus. Note the medial displacement of the temporal horn of the right lateral ventricle (*blue arrows*) and marked dilation of the left temporal horn (*green arrows*). Severe descending transtentorial herniation has resulted in compression of the contralateral left cerebral peduncle (*pink arrow*) against the medial left temporal lobe resulting in right hemiparesis. The resultant indentation of the left cerebral peduncle is known as Kernohan notch.

Postoperative Imaging of Subdural Hematomas

In the early postoperative period, noncontrast head CT is most commonly used to evaluate for potential complications. CT is widely available, fast, relatively inexpensive, and accurate at identifying most postoperative complications. Intracranial air in the early postoperative period can cause artifact on MRI. CT is sensitive for the identification of new intracranial hemorrhage, new mass effect and herniation, tension pneumocephalus, and calvarial fractures. Although MRI is less often used in the immediate postoperative period, it is much more sensitive for the detection of acute ischemia and infection. The choice to use MRI in the postoperative setting should be driven by the clinical scenario. If acute ischemia or infection is suspected clinically, MRI should always be considered.[1]

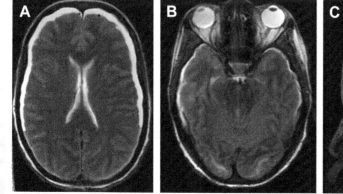
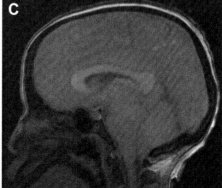

Fig. 35. MRI demonstrates bilateral subacute subdural hematomas (*A*) resulting in bilateral descending transtentorial (*B*) and acquired tonsillar herniation (*C*).

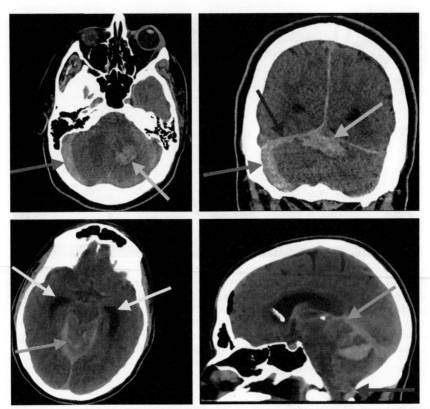

Fig. 36. Axial (*A, C*), coronal (*B*), and sagittal (*D*) NCCT demonstrates acute right posterior fossa subdural hematoma (*red arrows*) extending along the inferior right tentorial lealfet (*blue arrow*) and an acute parenchymal hematoma centrally in the cerebellum (*green arrows*). The posterior fossa hematoma results in ascending transtentorial (*orange arrows*) and early tonsillar herniation (*purple arrow*). Note how the superior cerebellar vermis fills the quadrigeminal and superior cerebellar cisterns, and compresses the dorsal midbrain. Also note the dilated temporal horns bilaterally caused by obstructive hydrocephalus at the level of the cerebral aqueduct/fourth ventricle (*yellow arrows*).

REFERENCES

1. Sinclair AG, Scoffings DJ. Imaging of the postoperative cranium. Radiographics 2010;30(2):461–82.
2. Dandy WE. Ventriculography following the injection of air into the cerebral ventricles. Ann Surg 1918; 68:5–11.
3. Pinto F. Ventriculography and pneumoencephalography; diagnosis of intracranial expansive processes. Rev Bras Cir 1957;33(5):506–9.
4. Antoni N. Cerebral herniations, their influence upon radiographic pictures, ventriculography and arteriography; a few anatomical specimens. Acta Psychiatr Neurol 1949;24(3–4):289–96.
5. Zaunbauer W. Multiple space-taking processes in cerebral roentgenography, with special reference to ventriculography. Wien Med Wochenschr 1952; 102(16):299–300 [in Undetermined Language].
6. White YS, Bell DS, Mellick R. Sequelae to pneumoencephalography. J Neurol Neurosurg Psychiatr 1973;36(1):146–51.
7. Rincon S, Gupta R, Ptak T. Imaging of head trauma. Handb Clin Neurol 2016;135:447–77.
8. Yamashima T, Friede RL. Why do bridging veins rupture into the virtual subdural space? J Neurol Neurosurg Psychiatr 1984;47(2):121–7.
9. Wintzen AR, Tijssen JG. Subdural hematoma and oral anticoagulant therapy. Arch Neurol 1982;39(2):69–72.
10. Boukas A, Sunderland GJ, Ross N. Prostate dural metastasis presenting as chronic subdural hematoma. A case report and review of the literature. Surg Neurol Int 2015;6:30.
11. Cheng CL, Greenberg J, Hoover LA. Prostatic adenocarcinoma metastatic to chronic subdural hematoma membranes. Case report. J Neurosurg 1988;68(4):642–4.
12. Beck J, Gralla J, Fung C, et al. Spinal cerebrospinal fluid leak as the cause of chronic subdural hematomas in nongeriatric patients. J Neurosurg 2014; 121(6):1380–7.
13. De noronha RJ, Sharrack B, Hadjivassiliou M, et al. Subdural haematoma: a potentially serious

consequence of spontaneous intracranial hypotension. J Neurol Neurosurg Psychiatr 2003; 74(6):752–5.

14. Wang HS, Kim SW, Kim SH. Spontaneous chronic subdural hematoma in an adolescent girl. J Korean Neurosurg Soc 2013;53(3):201–3.

15. Brennan PM, Fuller E, Shanmuganathan M, et al. Spontaneous subdural haematoma in a healthy young male. BMJ Case Rep 2011;2011.

16. Marconi F, Fiori L, Parenti G, et al. Acute spontaneous subdural haematoma. Description of four clinical cases. J Neurosurg Sci 1991;35(2):97–102.

17. Matsuda M, Matsuda I, Sato M, et al. Superior sagittal sinus thrombosis followed by subdural hematoma. Surg Neurol 1982;18:206–11.

18. Bansal H, Chaudhary A, Mahajan A, et al. Acute subdural hematoma secondary to cerebral venous sinus thrombosis: case report and review of literature. Asian J Neurosurg 2016;11(2):177.

19. Akins PT, Axelrod YK, Ji C, et al. Cerebral venous sinus thrombosis complicated by subdural hematomas: case series and literature review. Surg Neurol Int 2013;4:85.

20. Sahoo RK, Tripathy P, Praharaj HN. Cerebral venous sinus thrombosis with nontraumatic subdural hematoma. Int J Crit Illn Inj Sci 2015;5(1):59.

21. Byun HS, Patel PP. Spontaneous subdural hematoma of arterial origin: report of two cases. Neurosurgery 1979;5(5):611–3.

22. Guazzo EP, Xuereb JH. Spontaneous thrombosis of an arteriovenous malformation. J Neurol Neurosurg Psychiatr 1994;57(11):1410–2.

23. O'leary PM, Sweeny PJ. Ruptured intracerebral aneurysm resulting in a subdural hematoma. Ann Emerg Med 1986;15(8):944–6.

24. Mclaughlin MR, Jho HD, Kwon Y. Acute subdural hematoma caused by a ruptured giant intracavernous aneurysm: case report. Neurosurgery 1996;38(2): 388–92.

25. Kondziolka D, Bernstein M, Ter brugge K, et al. Acute subdural hematoma from ruptured posterior communicating artery aneurysm. Neurosurgery 1988;22(1 Pt 1):151–4.

26. Boujemâa H, Góngora-rivera F, Barragán-campos H, et al. Bilateral acute subdural hematoma from ruptured posterior communicating artery aneurysm. A case report. Interv Neuroradiol 2006;12(1): 37–40.

27. Scotti G, Terbrugge K, Melançon D, et al. Evaluation of the age of subdural hematomas by computerized tomography. J Neurosurg 1977;47(3):311–5.

28. Lee KS, Bae WK, Bae HG, et al. The computed tomographic attenuation and the age of subdural hematomas. J Korean Med Sci 1997;12(4):353–9.

29. Bradley WG. MR appearance of hemorrhage in the brain. Radiology 1993;189(1):15–26.

30. Gomori JM, Grossman RI. Mechanisms responsible for the MR appearance and evolution of intracranial hemorrhage. Radiographics 1988;8(3):427–40.

31. Fobben ES, Grossman RI, Atlas SW, et al. MR characteristics of subdural hematomas and hygromas at 1.5 T. AJR Am J Roentgenol 1989;153(3):589–95.

32. Gomori JM, Grossman RI, Bilaniuk LT, et al. High-field MR imaging of superficial siderosis of the central nervous system. J Comput Assist Tomogr 1985; 9(5):972–5.

33. Reed D, Robertson WD, Graeb DA, et al. Acute subdural hematomas: atypical CT findings. AJNR Am J Neuroradiol 1986;7(3):417–21.

34. Al-nakshabandi NA. The swirl sign. Radiology 2001; 218(2):433.

35. Smith WP, Batnitzky S, Rengachary SS. Acute iso-dense subdural hematomas: a problem in anemic patients. AJR Am J Roentgenol 1981;136(3):543–6.

36. Grelat M, Madkouri R, Bousquet O. Acute isodense subdural hematoma on computed tomography scan–diagnostic and therapeutic trap: a case report. J Med Case Rep 2016;10:43.

37. Wada R, Aviv RI, Fox AJ, et al. CT angiography "spot sign" predicts hematoma expansion in acute intracerebral hemorrhage. Stroke 2007;38(4):1257–62.

38. Markwalder TM. Chronic subdural hematomas: a review. J Neurosurg 1981;54(5):637–45.

39. Osborn AG. Osborn's brain, imaging, pathology, and anatomy. Lippincott Williams & Wilkins; 2012.

40. Hosoda K, Tamaki N, Masumura M, et al. Magnetic resonance images of chronic subdural hematomas. J Neurosurg 1987;67(5):677–83.

41. Lee KS, Shim JJ, Yoon SM, et al. Acute-on-chronic subdural hematoma: not uncommon events. J Korean Neurosurg Soc 2011;50(6):512–6.

42. Kloss BT, Lagace RE. Acute-on-chronic subdural hematoma. Int J Emerg Med 2010;3(4):511–2.

43. Tan S, Aronowitz P. Hematocrit effect in bilateral subdural hematomas. J Gen Intern Med 2013;28(2):321.

44. Bartels RH, Meijer FJ, Van der Hoeven H, et al. Midline shift in relation to thickness of traumatic acute subdural hematoma predicts mortality. BMC Neurol 2015;15:220.

45. Laine FJ, Shedden AI, Dunn MM, et al. Acquired intracranial herniations: MR imaging findings. AJR Am J Roentgenol 1995;165(4):967–73.

46. Osborn AG, Heaston DK, Wing SD. Diagnosis of ascending transtentorial herniation by cranial computed tomography. AJR Am J Roentgenol 1978;130(4):755–60.

Chronic Subdural Hematoma
Epidemiology and Natural History

Wuyang Yang, MD, MS, Judy Huang, MD*

KEYWORDS

- Chronic subdural hematoma • Epidemiology • Natural history • Pathogenesis

KEY POINTS

- Chronic subdural hematoma (CSDH) is a common disease that is prevalent predominantly in elderly patients.
- The incidence of CSDH ranges from 1.72 to 20.6 per 100,000 persons per year.
- Clinical progression of CSDH has 3 stages: initial formation, latency, and clinical presentation.
- Risk factors for CSDH include advancing age, male gender, and antiplatelet or anticoagulant use.

INTRODUCTION AND OVERVIEW

Chronic subdural hematoma (CSDH) is a common disease characterized by the abnormal collection of blood products in the subdural space with a relatively indolent course of disease progression.[1,2] The overall incidence of CSDH was reported to range from 1.72 to 20.6 per 100,000 persons per year,[3–8] with an incidence that is significantly higher in the elderly.[1,6,7,9] A trend toward an increase in incidence has been observed, and may be attributed to the overall aging population resulting from an increase in life expectancy.[10–12] The formation of CSDH remains unclear, and the pathophysiology has been hypothesized to be triggered by inflammatory responses,[13] transformation from acute subdural hematoma,[14] or an increased osmotic oncotic pressure gap between the hematoma and blood vessels.[15–17] Additionally, subclinical brain injury resulting in minor trauma to bridging veins may also facilitate the chronic accumulation of blood within the hematoma encapsulated by neomembranes.[11–14,18,19]

Manifestations of CSDH are variable, and mainly caused by immediate intracranial compression through expansion of the hematoma. Presenting symptoms include headaches, seizure, mental status changes, weakness, sensory disturbance, dysarthria, gait disturbance, nausea and vomiting, stroke, and coma.[20–22] In patients presenting with CSDH, 3% to 20% present with comatose status,[20,21,23,24] and severe impairment with brain herniation may occur in 2% of cases.[21] Of note, 10% to 30% of patients were also on anticoagulation or antiplatelet therapy.[10,12,23,25,26] CSDH can be diagnosed quickly using computed tomography, showing a crescent-shaped mass with a slight hypodensity representing the fluid sac of hematoma encased by the neomembranes.[27] Increased density and heterogeneous density may be noted as a natural progression of the disease or if recent bleeding is present.[28]

Disclosure Statement: The authors have nothing to disclose.
Department of Neurosurgery, Johns Hopkins University School of Medicine, 1800 Orleans Street, Zayed Tower, Suite 6115F, Baltimore, MD 21287, USA
* Corresponding author.
E-mail address: jhuang24@jhmi.edu

Neurosurg Clin N Am 28 (2017) 205–210
http://dx.doi.org/10.1016/j.nec.2016.11.002

Surgical evacuation of the hematoma remains the mainstay of treatment for symptomatic patients with diagnosed CSDH. Access to the hematoma capsule is approached through twist drill openings or burr hole openings; craniotomy is reserved generally for extensive hematoma, and is considered as a second-tier surgical option for most cases.[12,21,29,30] For asymptomatic patients, nonsurgical management is preferred, which includes eliminating precipitant factors such as anticoagulation or antiplatelet medications, correction of underlying coagulopathy, and symptom management.[12] Prognosis after surgical treatment has been favorable in most reported series, with 80% to 90% of treated patients achieving a satisfactory outcome at follow-up,[21] with mortality reported to be low at 0.5% to 4.3%.[20,21,23] Noticeably, the recurrence of CSDH may be as high as 70%, but only 10% to 20% of recurred CSDH require reoperation.[12,21,23,29,31–35]

EPIDEMIOLOGY

The incidence of CSDH has only been reported sporadically throughout the years. In a Finnish study conducted by Foelholm and Waltimo[4] in 1967, 64 residents of the city of Helsinki diagnosed with CSDH were included over a 7-year period, rendering an overall incidence of 1.72 per 100,000 persons per year. The authors highlighted a significant increase of incidence of up to 7.35 in the elderly population of 70 to 79 years of age. After this study, Kudo and colleagues[6] examined the incidence of CSDH in the Awaji island of Japan from 1986 to 1988, and concluded an overall incidence rate of 13.1 per 100,000 persons per year, with an incidence of 3.4 in the population under 65 years old and 58.1 in the elderly. A North Wales study by Asghar and colleagues[7] including patients between 1996 and 1999 revealed a lower incidence rate of 8.2 per 100,000 persons per year in patients greater than 65 years of age. In contrast, another Japanese study examining incidence of CSDH between 2005 and 2007 used data from a national registry. The authors reported an increased incidence of CSDH of 20.6 per 100,000 persons per year, with 76.5 in the 70 to 79 age group and 127.1 in the 80 years old age group.[3] Additionally, in a recent study by Balser and colleagues[8] focusing on the veteran population in United States, an overall incidence rate of 79.4 per 100,000 persons per year was observed, with age-standardized rate at 39.4 per 100,000 persons per year.

From these studies, it seems that the incidence of CSDH has been increasing over the years, with the increasing risk of CSDH attributable to the aging population and the increasing prevalence of anticoagulation/antiplatelet medication use in general populations.[3,4,6–9,12,13,24,25,27,28,33,35–38] However, the interpretation of the reported incidence rate should be managed with caution. To date, there are only 2 epidemiologic studies examining overall incidence of CSDH in a relatively closed population with low migration rates—the Finnish study and the Awaji island study in Japan—and a considerable difference in incidence rate has been noted between these 2 studies. Although the difference has been generally explained by increasing incidence of CSDH over the 20-year interval between these 2 studies,[8] the examined populations are heterogeneous, and confounding factors associated with population differences may also modify significantly the risk of CSDH. For instance, the incidence of traumatic brain injury, which is considered one of the precipitating factors for development of CSDH, is generally low in Finland, and may account for the lower rate of CSDH in the Finnish population. According to a nationwide, population-based study in Finland examining total traumatic brain injury from 1991 to 2005, the overall incidence was 101 per 100,000 persons per year, significantly lower than that reported in other countries, including the Netherlands, Estonia, and New Zealand.[39–42] In the veteran study where traumatic brain injury within the included population is considered highly prevalent, the projected incidence rate of CSDH was reported to be 121.4, which is significantly higher than that of the general population in other studies; conversely, in the same study, the prediction of CSDH incidence was only 17.4 in civilian-based models.[8] Additionally, in a study reported by Baechli and colleagues[37] examining the prevalence of CSDH in a large single-center study in Switzerland during a 7-year interval (1996–2002), the annual incidence remained relatively constant. Therefore, whether the global incidence of CSDH is truly increasing warrants cautious consideration, and the trend of an increased incidence for CSDH should be adjusted for population and environmental differences for accurate interpretation.

NATURAL HISTORY AND RISK FACTORS
Origin of Chronic Subdural Hematoma

Numerous theories have been proposed regarding the pathogenesis of CSDH. Virchow first related the origin of CSDH to an inflammatory response of the brain in 1857, in which he described a case of "pachymeningitis hemorrhagic interna," and noted a membranous structure in the inner surface of the dura believed to be the inflammatory origin for hematoma formation.[43,44] In contrast,

Trotter[45] favored a hematoma first etiology and suggested that the role of trauma in the development of CSDH. Putnam and Cushing, recalling a traumatic component in patients from both of their experiences, supported this theory by proposing the cause of CSDH to be originated from "an apparently insignificant trauma to the head," and indicated that the neomembranes formed in these cases "differs from that of the commonly described pachymeningitis hemorrhagica interna."[46] In a later review of the topic, Holmes[47] summarized all patients with diagnosis of CSDH in 3 Chicago hospitals between 1914 and 1925, and revealed that trauma is the factor in both cases of intraoperatively confirmed CSDH. The traumatic theory attributed the formation and expansion of hematoma to insignificant or repeated subclinical trauma. The fluid collection was hypothesized to be of vascular origin, either from transformation of asymptomatic acute hematoma, or microbleeding from neoformed vascular structures or torn bridging veins after trauma.

In contrast with theories suggesting the expansion of the hematoma through rupture of vessels, Gardner and Zollinger and their colleagues indicated that increased osmotic oncotic pressure owing to blood product breakdown within the hematoma capsule may be the major underlying mechanism for hematoma enlargement following initial hematoma formation.[15,17,48] However, this theory was not supported by later studies by Weir,[15,16] who noted no difference between the oncotic osmolality of subdural hematoma and cerebrospinal fluid or venous blood. Lee[14] also proposed that certain CSDHs may arise from incomplete resolution of acute subdural hematomas. In more recent studies, transformation of chronic subdural hygromas complicated with repeated ruptures in fragile neovascularized vessels into CSDH is believed to be the major pathway of CSDH formation.[14,19,28,49]

Clinical Progression of Chronic Subdural Hematoma

The clinical progression of CSDH can be generally categorized into 3 periods: the initial period of traumatic event, the latency period of hematoma expansion, and the clinical period of CSDH manifestation.[18,46] The initial period may present as either 1 or multiple clinical or subclinical traumatic events causing the initial formation of the hematoma, which is referred as the "seed" for CSDH development.[14] Immediately after the initial phase is the latent phase, in which the hematoma matures slowly and increases in volume. The neomembrane formation on the dural side as well as

on the arachnoid side facilitated the encapsulation of the hematoma, and was potentially the source of microhemorrhages owing to fragility of vessels formed by extensive neovascularization.[28] The hyperactivation of the fibrinolytic system has also been proposed to play a role in the extension of hematoma.[31] During this period, patients may be asymptomatic, and this may last for weeks to years.[14,46,50,51] After the latency period, progressive decompensation of intracranial capacity occurs as a result of continuous growing of the hematoma capsule, and a constellation of symptoms may appear from increased intracranial pressure.[18] At clinical presentation, approximately 10% to 20% present with seizures,[20,23] 2% to 15% with coma, and 2% with brain herniation.[20,21,24] Of note, less than 1% of all reported cases were discovered incidentally.[10,20,24] Without any treatment, few CSDHs have been reported to regress spontaneously,[52,53] whereas 40% of all patients may eventually recover on medical management without surgical intervention. However, 20% of patients undergoing conservative management experience clinical deterioration and require surgical intervention.[54]

Risk Factors for Chronic Subdural Hematoma

It is evident in the literature that CSDH is not a static disease, and the risk of development, progression, and recurrence of CSDH may be modified significantly by several risk factors. Among all risk factors identified to date, the association of older age with risk of CSDH occurrence has been consistently described by existing literature.[1,6,7,9] Epidemiologic studies reported significant increase in incidence of CSDH in the elderly compared with other age cohorts[3,6,8]; in addition, most CSDH case series also reported their cohort to be composed of patients with advanced age at mean age of 55 to 60 years, with some greater than 70 years of age.[10,22–24,37] The underlying reason for greater prevalence of CSDH among the elderly is not completely understood, but may be attributed to a higher risk of falls in this population. In a study conducted by Baechli and coauthors[37] including 354 consecutive CSDH patients, 69% of all patients were more than 65 year os age, and falls were reported in 77% of the cohort. Although the authors highlighted a trend toward a greater risk of falls in the elderly with a relative risk of 1.11, however, the result did not attain significance.[37]

Male gender was also recognized to be a potential risk factor for CSDH. The Finnish epidemiologic study on the incidence of CSDH demonstrated an overall higher incidence for men over women. This trend was unchanged in the same cohort after stratification by age.[4] Similarly, a male gender predominance of the incidence and prevalence of the disease was also observed in other CSDH studies.[1,3,6,7,9,10,13,20,23,24,28,37,51,55] The difference in gender distribution of CSDH might not be related to falls; in 1 study, the risk of fall was reported to be similar between the 2 gender groups. However, the authors also noted that male gender may have been more likely to be exposed to injuries or other CSDH-related factors in general.[37] This assumption is corroborated by discovery of CSDH-associated factors with a known male predominance, such as alcohol use and epilepsy.[11] Male gender was also reported to bear a higher rate of recurrence after treatment for CSDH.[22]

Aside from demographic risk factors, anticoagulation or antiplatelet therapy was also considered a risk factor for occurrence, as well as recurrence of CSDH. Because most patients with CSDH were elderly, an increased proportion of patients on anticoagulant agents for the prevention or treatment of systemic diseases is superimposed. Rust and colleagues[36] observed 81 cases of CSDH in 2001 and 2002 within a defined population of 460,000 to 473,252 in Tasmania, Australia. The total number of patients taking warfarin in both years were collected from national insurance database, and the incidence of CSDH in patients on warfarin was noted to be 0.08% to 0.40% per year, compared with 0.002% to 0.010% per year in those without warfarin, rendering a greater than 40 times higher risk of CSDH development in warfarin users. Besides occurrence of CSDH, both anticoagulant and antiplatelet agents were also proposed to be associated potentially with the expansion of hematoma.[32] The association of both medications with recurrence of CSDH was less clear and has been reported to be irrelevant in many studies.[11,32,56]

RECURRENCE

Although surgical treatment using the twist drill or burr hole techniques have been shown to be effective in the management of CSDH,[21,29,33,35] recurrence still occurs in a small portion of the treated patients. The risk of recurrence in a surgical series was reported to be 3% to 20% in different study populations with burr hole techniques.[23,28] In contrast, for patients undergoing craniectomy, the recurrence rate was noted to be significantly lower.[20] Interestingly, the recurrence rate for CSDH patients who were managed conservatively was also low. Suzuki and colleagues[57] found no occurrence in their case series of 23 patients undergoing conservative management, and they further noted that complete clinical recovery was achieved in 22 patients with only mannitol administration. Similarly, Kageyama and coauthors[31] described using tranexamic acid as the only therapy in 18 patients, and no recurrence of hematoma was observed. In a review of reported cases by Horikoshi and colleagues,[58] the rate of spontaneous resolution of CSDH with or without medical therapy is approximately 2.4% to 18.5%. The risk of recurrence varies greatly among different treatment strategies, and might be an indication of effectiveness of the management strategy; however, provided that a strong tendency for surgical intervention is implied in emergency cases, the difference of recurrence risk in management arms is more likely to be reflective of a selection bias.

A variety of nonsurgical risk factors has been proposed to be associated with recurrence of CSDH, this included elderly age, patient status on admission, alcohol consumption, systemic diseases such as renal and liver dysfunction, and bilateral CSDH.[23] As mentioned, the role of anticoagulant or antiplatelet medication use in the recurrence of CSDH is controversial. The location and lesion architecture of CSDH was also noted to modify the risk of recurrence. In a study of 106 CSDH patients conducted by Nakaguchi and colleagues,[28] a staging system based on computed tomography appearance was proposed, and the association between different lesion stages and rate of recurrence was emphasized. The authors noted a higher recurrence in the "separated type" and lower recurrence in the "trabeculated type"; cranial base CSDH was also noted to be associated significantly with recurrence than convexity types.

SUMMARY

Despite being a long-standing disease, many aspects of epidemiology and natural history of CSDH remains to be elucidated. The overall incidence rate has been reported to be 1.72% to 20.6% per 100,000 persons per year in the general population, and more commonly affecting the elderly. Despite an increasing trend in the reported incidence of CSDH, the heterogeneity of study populations renders a difficult comparison across these studies, and further investigation of incidence rate adjusted by risk factors on a population scale is warranted for accurate interpretation. A variety of mechanisms of CSDH development have been proposed, including inflammatory mechanisms, increased oncotic osmolality pressure, incomplete resolution from acute subdural hemorrhage, and microbleeding from repeated trauma. Although spontaneous CSDH resolution occurs, most patients require surgical evacuation of the hematoma for an optimal clinical outcome. Multiple risk factors may modify the risk of CSDH development and progression, including elderly age and male gender. The increasing use of anticoagulants and antiplatelet medications was also associated with hematoma progression and expansion in CSDH patients. Recurrence of CSDH after treatment may occur in 3% to 20% of all treated patients. Although a lower rate was found in patients managed conservatively, selection of high-risk patients for surgical intervention is likely to account for the differences in recurrence rates.

REFERENCES

1. Miranda LB, Braxton E, Hobbs J, et al. Chronic subdural hematoma in the elderly: not a benign disease. J Neurosurg 2011;114(1):72–6.
2. Maurice-Williams RS. Chronic subdural haematoma: an everyday problem for the neurosurgeon. Br J Neurosurg 1999;13(6):547–9.
3. Karibe H, Kameyama M, Kawase M, et al. Epidemiology of chronic subdural hematomas. No Shinkei Geka 2011;39(12):1149–53 [in Japanese].
4. Foelholm R, Waltimo O. Epidemiology of chronic subdural haematoma. Acta Neurochir (Wien) 1975; 32(3–4):247–50.
5. Sarti C, Tuomilehto J, Salomaa V, et al. Epidemiology of subarachnoid hemorrhage in Finland from 1983 to 1985. Stroke 1991;22(7):848–53.
6. Kudo H, Kuwamura K, Izawa I, et al. Chronic subdural hematoma in elderly people: present status on Awaji Island and epidemiological prospect. Neurol Med Chir (Tokyo) 1992;32(4):207–9.
7. Asghar M, Adhiyaman V, Greenway MW, et al. Chronic subdural haematoma in the elderly–a North Wales experience. J R Soc Med 2002;95(6):290–2.
8. Balser D, Farooq S, Mehmood T, et al. Actual and projected incidence rates for chronic subdural hematomas in United States veterans administration and civilian populations. J Neurosurg 2015;123(5): 1209–15.
9. Adhiyaman V, Asghar M, Ganeshram KN, et al. Chronic subdural haematoma in the elderly. Postgrad Med J 2002;78(916):71–5.
10. Farhat Neto J, Araujo JLV, Ferraz VR, et al. Chronic subdural hematoma: epidemiological and prognostic analysis of 176 cases. Rev Col Bras Cir 2015;42(5):283–7.
11. Santarius T, Kirkpatrick PJ, Kolias AG, et al. Working toward rational and evidence-based treatment of chronic subdural hematoma. Clin Neurosurg 2010; 57:112–22.
12. Kolias AG, Chari A, Santarius T, et al. Chronic subdural haematoma: modern management and emerging therapies. Nat Rev Neurol 2014;10(10): 570–8.
13. Chen JC, Levy ML. Causes, epidemiology, and risk factors of chronic subdural hematoma. Neurosurg Clin N Am 2000;11(3):399–406.
14. Lee K-S. Natural history of chronic subdural haematoma. Brain Inj 2004;18(4):351–8.
15. Weir B. The osmolality of subdural hematoma fluid. J Neurosurg 1971;34(4):528–33.
16. Weir B. Oncotic pressure of subdural fluids. J Neurosurg 1980;53(4):512–5.
17. Zollinger R, Gross RE. Traumatic subdural hematoma. JAMA 1934;103(4):245–9.
18. Iliescu IA, Constantinescu AI. Clinical evolutional aspects of chronic subdural haematomas - literature review. J Med Life 2015;8(Spec Issue):26–33.
19. Lee K-S. History of chronic subdural hematoma. Korean J Neurotrauma 2015;11(2):27–34.
20. Sambasivan M. An overview of chronic subdural hematoma: experience with 2300 cases. Surg Neurol 1997;47(5):418–22.
21. Mori K, Maeda M. Surgical treatment of chronic subdural hematoma in 500 consecutive cases: clinical characteristics, surgical outcome, complications, and recurrence rate. Neurol Med Chir (Tokyo) 2001;41(8):371–81.
22. Kim J, Moon J, Kim T, et al. Risk factor analysis for the recurrence of chronic subdural hematoma: a review of 368 consecutive surgical cases. Korean J Neurotrauma 2015;11(2):63–9.
23. Gelabert-González M, Iglesias-Pais M, García-Allut A, et al. Chronic subdural haematoma: surgical treatment and outcome in 1000 cases. Clin Neurol Neurosurg 2005;107(3):223–9.
24. Cameron MM. Chronic subdural haematoma: a review of 114 cases. J Neurol Neurosurg Psychiatr 1978;41(9):834–9.
25. Aspegren OP, Åstrand R, Lundgren MI, et al. Anticoagulation therapy a risk factor for the development of chronic subdural hematoma. Clin Neurol Neurosurg 2013;115(7):981–4.
26. Mellergård P, Wisten O. Operations and reoperations for chronic subdural haematomas during a 25-year period in a well defined population. Acta Neurochir (Wien) 1996;138(6):708–13.
27. Tanaka Y, Ohno K. Chronic subdural hematoma - an up-to-date concept. J Med Dent Sci 2013;60(2):55–61.
28. Nakaguchi H, Tanishima T, Yoshimasu N. Factors in the natural history of chronic subdural hematomas that influence their postoperative recurrence. J Neurosurg 2001;95(2):256–62.
29. Ivamoto HS, Lemos HP, Atallah AN. Surgical treatments for chronic subdural hematomas: a comprehensive systematic review. World Neurosurg 2016; 86:399–418.
30. Weigel R, Schmiedek P, Krauss JK. Outcome of contemporary surgery for chronic subdural haematoma: evidence based review. J Neurol Neurosurg Psychiatr 2003;74(7):937–43.

31. Kageyama H, Toyooka T, Tsuzuki N, et al. Nonsurgical treatment of chronic subdural hematoma with tranexamic acid. J Neurosurg 2013;119(2):332–7.

32. Torihashi K, Sadamasa N, Yoshida K, et al. Independent predictors for recurrence of chronic subdural hematoma: a review of 343 consecutive surgical cases. Neurosurgery 2008;63(6):1125–9 [discussion: 1129].

33. Ducruet AF, Grobelny BT, Zacharia BE, et al. The surgical management of chronic subdural hematoma. Neurosurg Rev 2012;35(2):155–69 [discussion: 169].

34. Guha D, Coyne S, MacDonald RL. Timing of the resumption of antithrombotic agents following surgical evacuation of chronic subdural hematomas: a retrospective cohort study. J Neurosurg 2016; 124(3):750–9.

35. Liu W, Bakker NA, Groen RJM. Chronic subdural hematoma: a systematic review and meta-analysis of surgical procedures. J Neurosurg 2014;121(3): 665–73.

36. Rust T, Kiemer N, Erasmus A. Chronic subdural haematomas and anticoagulation or anti-thrombotic therapy. J Clin Neurosci 2006;13(8):823–7.

37. Baechli H, Nordmann A, Bucher HC, et al. Demographics and prevalent risk factors of chronic subdural haematoma: results of a large single-center cohort study. Neurosurg Rev 2004;27(4):263–6.

38. Markwalder TM. Chronic subdural hematomas: a review. J Neurosurg 1981;54(5):637–45.

39. Koskinen S, Alaranta H. Traumatic brain injury in Finland 1991-2005: a nationwide register study of hospitalized and fatal TBI. Brain Inj 2008;22(3): 205–14.

40. Scholten AC, Haagsma JA, Panneman MJM, et al. Traumatic brain injury in the Netherlands: incidence, costs and disability-adjusted life years. PLoS One 2014;9(10):e110905.

41. Ventsel G, Kolk A, Talvik I, et al. The incidence of childhood traumatic brain injury in Tartu and Tartu County in Estonia. Neuroepidemiology 2008; 30(1):20–4.

42. Feigin VL, Theadom A, Barker-Collo S, et al. Incidence of traumatic brain injury in New Zealand: a population-based study. Lancet Neurol 2013;12(1): 53–64.

43. Virchow R. Das Ha'matom der dura mater. Verh Phys Med Ges 1857;7:134–42.

44. Schwartz AB. The etiology of pachymeningitis hemorrhagica interna in infants. Arch Pediatr Adolesc Med 1916;XI(1):23–32.

45. Trotter W. Chronic subdural haemorrhage of traumatic origin, and its relation to pachymeningitis hemorrhagica interna. Br J Surg 1914;2:271–91.

46. Putnam TJ. Chronic subdural hematoma. Arch Surg 1925;11(3):329–93.

47. Holmes WH. Chronic subdural hematoma. Arch Neurpsych 1928;20(1):162–70.

48. Gardner WJ. Traumatic subdural hematoma. Arch Neurpsych 1932;27(4):847–58.

49. Lee K-S, Bae WK, Doh JW, et al. Origin of chronic subdural haematoma and relation to traumatic subdural lesions. Brain Inj 1998;12(11):901–10.

50. Kotwica Z, Brzeziński J. A long course of chronic subdural haematomas. Acta Neurochir (Wien) 1987;85(1–2):44–5.

51. Liliang P-C, Tsai Y-D, Liang C-L, et al. Chronic subdural haematoma in young and extremely aged adults: a comparative study of two age groups. Injury 2002;33(4):345–8.

52. Parlato C, Guarracino A, Moraci A. Spontaneous resolution of chronic subdural hematoma. Surg Neurol 2000;53(4):312–5 [discussion: 315–7].

53. Naganuma H, Fukamachi A, Kawakami M, et al. Spontaneous resolution of chronic subdural hematomas. Neurosurgery 1986;19(5):794–8.

54. Bender MB, Christoff N. Nonsurgical treatment of subdural hematomas. Arch Neurol 1974;31(2):73–9.

55. Almenawer SA, Farrokhyar F, Hong C, et al. Chronic subdural hematoma management: a systematic review and meta-analysis of 34,829 patients. Ann Surg 2014;259(3):449–57.

56. Gonugunta V, Buxton N. Warfarin and chronic subdural haematomas. Br J Neurosurg 2001;15(6): 514–7.

57. Suzuki J, Takaku A. Nonsurgical treatment of chronic subdural hematoma. J Neurosurg 1970;33(5):548–53.

58. Horikoshi T, Naganuma H, Fukasawa I, et al. Computed tomography characteristics suggestive of spontaneous resolution of chronic subdural hematoma. Neurol Med Chir (Tokyo) 1998;38(9):527–32 [discussion: 532–3].

Chronic Subdural Medical Management

David Roh, MD*, Michael Reznik, MD, Jan Claassen, MD, PhD

KEYWORDS

- Subdural hematoma • Medical management • Nonoperative • Antiepileptic drug • Steroid
- HMG-CoA reductase inhibitor • Angiotensin-converting enzyme inhibitor • Antifibrinolytic

KEY POINTS

- Prophylactic antiepileptic medication use is recommended for patients with symptomatic, chronic subdural hematomas (cSDHs) deemed at high risk for seizure.
- Both asymptomatic and, mildly symptomatic, good grade cSDH may be amenable to nonoperative medical management.
- Steroid therapy decreases inflammatory mechanisms that contribute to hyperpermeability and angiogenesis in cSDH, and has evidence for a role in nonoperative, medical management of cSDH.
- 3-Hydroxy-3-methylglutaryl-coenzyme A reductase inhibitors, angiotensin-converting enzyme inhibitors, and antifibrinolytic agents are other proposed medical treatments to cSDH that require further study.

INTRODUCTION

Chronic subdural hematoma (cSDH), which is characterized by a time course of weeks to months, has become an increasingly detected neurosurgical disease. This increased prevalence can be attributed in part to a growing aging population and increased antithrombotic medication use. However, uniform consensus guidelines are lacking because of the heterogeneity of both the disease and the collection of data and outcomes surrounding it. Surgical drainage via burr-hole craniostomy has been the mainstay of treatment of symptomatic cSDH, but conservative management options are considered in those patients who have asymptomatic, small-volume cSDH, or for those in whom surgery carries a high risk. This article focuses on the current practices, potential strategies, and evidence for the medical management of cSDHs.

PATIENT EVALUATION OVERVIEW

cSDH is an increasingly detected disease in the elderly, with estimates of about 10 per 100,000 a year[1] (further details on epidemiology, pathophysiology, and history of cSDH are presented elsewhere). Presentations can vary widely ranging from mild symptoms of headaches or subtle behavioral changes to more clinically significant symptoms of focal weakness, gait disturbance, seizures, or decreased mental status. These symptoms are often gradual and can be progressive over a course of days to weeks. A preceding history of head trauma may be either minor or absent in cases of cSDH.

The preferred imaging modality is a computed tomography (CT) scan with a hematoma appearance that can range from isodense (30–60 Hounsfield units) to hypodense (<30 Hounsfield units); the transition from the hyperdense appearance of an acute hematoma to that of a cSDH typically

Disclosure: Dr D. Roh and M. Reznik have nothing to disclose. Dr J. Claassen has served on the Advisory Board for study planning at SAGE pharmaceuticals, Actelion, and BARD pharmaceuticals.
Department of Neurology, Columbia University Medical Center, 177 Fort Washington Avenue, Milstein Building 8GS-300, New York, NY 10032, USA
* Corresponding author.
E-mail address: dr2753@cumc.columbia.edu

Neurosurg Clin N Am 28 (2017) 211–217
http://dx.doi.org/10.1016/j.nec.2016.11.003
1042-3680/17/© 2016 Elsevier Inc. All rights reserved.

neurosurgery.theclinics.com

occurs after 3 weeks. It is unclear if clinical and radiographic characteristics can determine the progression and subsequent of cSDH. However, some cohort studies have shown that worse admission Glasgow Coma Scale (GCS) and modified Rankin Scale (mRS) scores may be associated with worse outcomes.[2,3] To be able to better characterize the clinical grades of patients with cSDH, the Markwalder score was created. Higher grades were associated with lower rates of perioperative brain expansion in the original study (**Table 1**).[4] This scoring system is now primarily used as a tool to evaluate the clinical severity of cSDH, with higher scores being associated with more severe injury. Neuroimaging characteristics, particularly the size of the hematoma, may be associated with outcome as small, asymptomatic cSDHs may spontaneously resolve and be associated with better outcomes.

cSDH has been associated with lower mortality compared with acute subdural hematoma (SDH). Early literature quoted low mortality rates of 2.8% for patients with cSDH who received surgery[5] compared with widely ranging rates of 40% to 90% in patients with acute SDH receiving surgery.[6] However, lengths of follow-up for the patients with cSDH in these initial reviews were unclear, and subsequent retrospective follow-up studies found much higher rates of mortality in surgically treated cSDH: 16% on discharge and 32% at 1 year.[7] This evidence revealed that cSDH is not a benign disease and has supported the widespread practice of surgical intervention with evidence of favorable outcomes after surgery.

Alternatively, because cSDH is increasingly detected in patients with minimal or no symptoms, invasive surgical treatments may not be the best approach in all cases. Previously utilized, conservative watch-and-wait approaches have been suboptimal, because many of these conservatively managed patients gradually develop symptoms and continue to have expansion of their cSDH that necessitates surgery. However, evidence is now emerging for initial conservative measures involving medical management for patients with asymptomatic or low-grade small-volume cSDH, or for those in whom surgery poses great risk. Regardless of the selection of treatment (whether it be surgical or medical), close follow-up of these patients is paramount; although cSDH was once thought to be benign, it is now known to be associated with mortality both during hospitalization and after discharge.

ANTIEPILEPTIC USE

A cornerstone of medical management in this patient population is the prevention and treatment of seizures. However, studies investigating the role for prophylactic antiepileptic drugs (AEDs) in cSDH have had mixed results, preventing guidelines from making high-level recommendations due to a lack of class I evidence. It is still common practice to start patients with cSDH on prophylactic AEDs, most likely because of the high rates of seizures reported in older literature. However, closer evaluation reveals that the incidence of seizures varies widely from one study to another, with a range from 2% to 17%[8] and increasing to up to 23% postoperatively.[9] This variability most likely stems from heterogeneous cSDH severity and differences in surgical treatment. Meanwhile, the incidence of seizures in nonoperative, spontaneously resolving cSDH is unknown.

Although the necessity of treating seizures in the setting of cSDH is clear, the utility of prophylactic AEDs depends on appropriate patient selection; patients with cSDH are more likely to be vulnerable to side effects of AEDs given their older age, and any benefit may therefore be offset by these risks. There have been no comparative randomized controlled trials that address this issue, although there are several retrospective studies on the role of prophylactic AEDs that have yielded mixed results. A retrospective Japanese review of 129 patients with cSDH revealed a low preoperative seizure rate of 1% in its population (N = 2; both in nonprophylactic group). There were 73 patients who received prophylactic AEDs (phenobarbital) and 56 who did not. Postoperatively, only 2 patients developed seizures, with both patients being in the nonprophylactic AED group; however, both were thought to be related to surgical technique and severity of injury. As a result, the investigators

Table 1 Markwalder Score for cSDH	
Grade 0	Asymptomatic
Grade 1	Alert, oriented, mild symptoms
Grade 2	Drowsy or disoriented, variable neurologic deficits
Grade 3	Stuporous but responding appropriately to noxious stimuli, severe focal signs
Grade 4	Comatose, absent motor response to painful stimuli, decerebrate or decorticate posturing

From Markwalder TM, Steinsiepe KF, Rohner M, et al. The course of chronic subdural hematomas after burr-hole craniostomy and closed-system drainage. J Neurosurg 1981;55:391; with permission.

concluded that AED prophylaxis should only be considered in patients with cSDH with extensive injury burden.[8] Similarly, another retrospective cohort analysis on 138 patients revealed that, of the 83 patients who received prophylactic AEDs, 4 (4.5%) developed seizures, whereas only 2 of 55 (3.4%) patients not treated with AEDs developed seizures.[10]

An additional retrospective analysis of 98 patients with cSDH revealed that only 1 patient of 42 (2.4%) who received prophylactic AED (phenytoin) developed seizures compared with 16 of 50 (32%) in those that did not receive prophylaxis. Seizures were associated with increased morbidity and mortality, suggesting the potential importance of prophylactic AEDs for surgical patients with cSDH.[11] A more recent retrospective cohort analysis revealed that, out of 88 patients with cSDH, 60 (71%) received preoperative prophylactic AEDs, and these significantly reduced the incidence of postoperative seizures compared with patients who received AED prophylaxis postoperatively. This finding suggests that timing of the initiation of prophylactic AEDs preoperatively may also be important.[9]

Additional studies have attempted to characterize seizure risk based on neuroimaging characteristics, with high-risk patients having cSDH with mixed densities and membranes.[12] Furthermore, the locale of SDH also plays a role in the epileptogenic potential, with the temporal lobe being particularly prone. However, most of these studies have been performed on patients with cSDH who ultimately require surgery. The incidence of seizures remains unclear for the subset of patients in whom the cSDH may resolve on its own. Even more questions arise in selecting the appropriate AED for seizure prophylaxis, although levetiracetam seems to be increasingly preferred because of a favorable side effect profile compared with traditionally used phenytoin.[13,14]

Although the role of anticonvulsants in cSDH requires further study, current recommendations call for prophylactic AEDs to be used for cSDH at high risk for seizures with caution for the potential harm of associated side effects with these medications. Considerations for patients deemed to be at high risk for developing seizures can be made for those who have some of the following characteristics (Table 2): history of alcohol abuse, clinical presentation of altered mental status/low GCS score, neuroimaging characteristics with significant underlying brain injury, evidence of mixed densities of blood and membranes, and in circumstances in which the primary blood burden is in epileptogenic regions (eg, temporal lobe).

Table 2
Suggested indications and medication use for prophylactic antiepileptic treatment in chronic subdural hematoma

Suggested indications for prophylactic AED	Clinical: • History of ethyl alcohol abuse • Altered mental status • GCS <9 Imaging: • Significant underlying brain injury • Mixed densities of blood and presence of membranes • Location of bleed near epileptogenic regions (temporal lobe, tentorium)
Suggested prophylactic AED use	Levetiracetam Valproic acid if significant behavioral/psychiatric issues

CORTICOSTEROIDS

The pathophysiology of cSDH (discussed in detail in chapter 2) is thought to be multifactorial. One component is the existence of a localized inflammatory reaction following cSDH as a result of a disruption of dural border cells.[15,16] This localized inflammatory reaction may promote angiogenesis and hyperpermeability,[17] leading to propagation of ongoing bleeding. The use of corticosteroids for medical management of cSDH has been thought to address and limit local inflammation and angiogenesis. Initial reports of successful conservative medical management strategies have led to increasing evidence in both retrospective and prospective series (Table 3) that steroids may have a role in certain cases of cSDH, particularly when surgery is not an option.

In a retrospective analysis of a prospectively studied, single-center cohort of 112 patients with cSDH, 26 patients with lower grade cSDH received medical treatment with dexamethasone (16 mg/d for 21 days). The dexamethasone-treated patients had comparable outcomes/mortalities with those who received surgery, although this was limited by extensive inpatient stay compared with the surgical group.[18] A subsequent retrospective study found that, of 122 consecutive patients with cSDH, 101 received dexamethasone (12 mg/d for 2–3 days followed by slow taper).

Table 3
Studies of nonsurgical management in chronic subdural hematomas (excluding case reports and studies of surgery with adjunctive medical treatment)

Investigators (Year)	Study Type	Treated Patients	Treatment	Outcome
Sun et al,[18] 2005	Prospective	26	Dexamethasone (16 mg/d for 21 d)	• 1 patient required subsequent surgery • 1 patient died • 22 patients with good neurologic outcome
Delgado-Lopez et al,[19] 2009	Retrospective	101	Dexamethasone (12 mg/d for 2–3 d followed by slow tapering)	• 22 patients required subsequent surgery • 1 patient died • 97 patients with good neurologic outcome
Thotakura & Marabathina,[20] 2015	Prospective	26	Dexamethasone (12 mg/d for 3 d followed by a 1-mo oral taper)	• 15 patients required subsequent surgery • 0 patients died • 26 patients with good neurologic outcome
Prud'homme et al,[21] 2016	Prospective, randomized, placebo controlled	20	Dexamethasone (12 mg/d for 3 wk followed by tapering) or placebo	• 1 patient in steroid group and 3 patients in placebo group required subsequent surgery • 2 patients in steroid group and 0 patients in placebo group died • Outcomes not assessed
Li et al,[30] 2014	Prospective	23	Atorvastatin (20 mg/d for 1–6 mo)	• 1 patient required subsequent surgery • 0 patients died • 22 patients with good neurologic outcome
Kageyama et al,[34] 2013	Retrospective	21	Tranexamic acid (750 mg/d until resolution)	• No hematoma progression • 3 out of 21 patients required surgery (not related to hemorrhage expansion) • No comparator group • No thromboembolic complications

Dexamethasone treatment was assigned to patients with low-grade cSDH, of whom 22 (21.8%) ultimately required surgical drainage. Outcomes were favorable in both surgical and dexamethasone groups, potentially suggesting a role for treatment with dexamethasone only in patients with lower grade cSDH.[19]

A more recent, single-center prospective study treated 26 patients with cSDH with GCS 15 with intravenous (IV) dexamethasone 12 mg/d for 3 days (with a 1-month oral taper thereafter). A standard burr-hole evacuation was done only if the patient had not improved by 3 days. Of these patients, 11 were treated successfully with steroids, whereas 15 required surgery, with female sex, less midline shift, and density (in Hounsfield units) associated with successful medical treatment.[20]

In addition, a small, single-center, placebo-controlled, prospective trial randomized 20 patients with no more than mild-moderate symptoms to receive dexamethasone 12 mg/d for 3 weeks (followed by tapering) or placebo, and then followed them for 6 months. Of these patients, 1 out of 10 in the steroid group and 3 out of 10 in the placebo group had to undergo surgical drainage, whereas the remainder of patients had complete radiologic resolution. Side effects were subjectively assessed via patient questionnaires, and the investigators noted that there was the suggestion of more subjective adverse events in the dexamethasone group.[21]

The role of steroids as an adjunct to surgical treatment has also been studied. A retrospective study of 198 consecutive patients with cSDH over 4 years revealed that 142 received corticosteroids (oral prednisolone or IV methylprednisolone at 0.5 mg/kg for 24 hours) as an adjunct to operative management. These patients had a significantly higher rate of survival than patients who did not receive steroids.[22] An additional retrospective study of 496 consecutive patients with cSDH over 18 years who were treated with burr-hole craniotomy and adjunctive dexamethasone showed that longer perioperative dexamethasone treatment was associated with a lower risk of SDH recurrence.[3]

In practice, the use of steroids seems to have become more common but has yet to become widespread and has differed across not only the United states, but the world. Rates of steroid use in cSDH have ranged from 13% to 55% in conservatively managed patients.[23–25] Despite the recent accumulation of supporting evidence for the use of corticosteroids, whether used as perioperative adjuvant therapy or as monotherapy, more high-quality studies are needed to further affect clinical practice. Clinical trials are currently ongoing to better establish evidence for their use, especially given the potential for side effects in an at-risk elderly population. Such side effects may include delirium, bone fractures, and infection. Given these risks, further investigations are also ongoing with antiinflammatory agents that may be better tolerated in an elderly population.

3-HYDROXY-3-METHYLGLUTARYL-COENZYME A REDUCTASE INHIBITOR (STATIN)

Corticosteroids have become an emerging treatment of cSDH and, for many of the same reasons, studies have explored the use of 3-hydroxy-3-methylglutaryl-coenzyme A (HMG-CoA) reductase inhibitors. Aside from their lipid level–lowering effects, statins have been shown to have potent systemic antiinflammatory properties.[26] Studies have suggested that statins also promote angiogenesis,[27–29] but the extent to which angiogenesis may either exacerbate or temper recurrent bleeding is unclear. At this time, evidence to support HMG-CoA reductase inhibitors in cSDH is limited to animal models and 1 small clinical study.

In a rat model of SDH, treatment with atorvastatin at 3 mg/kg/d for 7 days was compared with placebo and the decrease in hematoma volume at day 7 was significantly greater in the atorvastatin group. This was also accompanied by a greater improvement in neurological outcome.[30] Further microscopic and immunohistochemical analysis revealed that the atorvastatin group had significantly lower levels of neutrophilic granulocytes and lower levels of tumor necrosis factor alpha and interleulin-6 in the SDH neomembrane, which the investigators attributed to attenuated inflammatory response leading to decreased SDH volumes.

A subsequent multicenter pilot study followed 23 patients with good-grade cSDHs (Markwalder score 0–3) who received oral atorvastatin at a dose of 20 mg/d for 1 to 6 months.[27] Of these patients, 1 patient required surgery because of clinical deterioration and hematoma enlargement after 4 weeks, whereas the other 22 experienced an improvement in their symptoms. Hematomas completely resolved in 17 patients by 3 months, and none of the 22 nonsurgical patients had a relapse during the follow-up period (which ranged from 3–36 months).

Given the limited data available for statin therapy in cSDHs, more evidence is needed before statins can be recommended in clinical practice. However, preliminary data seem promising for those patients in whom surgical intervention may not be an option. Enrollment for a prospective randomized controlled trial is currently ongoing.[23]

ANGIOTENSIN-CONVERTING ENZYME INHIBITORS AND ANTIFIBRINOLYTIC AGENTS

Given the aforementioned pathophysiologic inflammatory mechanisms of cSDH formation and growth, angiotensin-converting enzyme inhibitors (ACEi) have been thought to have an antiangiogenic effect via tempering of the vascular endothelial growth factor (VEGF) expression that is thought to precipitate further bleeding in cSDH. An initial retrospective study of 310 patients with operative cSDH compared ACEi users and non–ACEi users. Although the doses and ACEi types were not specified, the ACEi group seemed to have significantly lower rates of SDH recurrence (5% vs 18%, along with improved outcomes) and lower hematoma concentrations of VEGF, suggesting a role for ACEi for medical management of cSDH.[31] Although, these results were initially promising, follow-up studies have failed to replicate these findings.[32,33]

Hyperfibrinolysis is also thought to occur in cSDH, thereby potentiating liquefaction of the hematoma and causing cSDH expansion. Consequently, antifibrinolytics have been studied as potential agents in the medical management of cSDH. To date, only 1 retrospective cohort study from Japan has studied the impact of tranexamic acid on medical management of cSDH. In this study, 21 patients were treated with oral tranexamic acid (750 mg daily, until hematoma resolution) for their cSDH regardless of symptoms or surgical intervention.[34] Of these patients, 18 (86%) received tranexamic acid only without surgery and all 21 patients in the cohort had decreased cSDH size (compared with historical rates of resolution in nontreated cSDH of 2%–18%). Treatment day ranges were widely variable (28–137 days), and it is unclear whether the rates of cSDH resolution reflected the natural course of cSDH. However, this study showed that there were no adverse side effects despite the prolonged course of antifibrinolytic therapy.

SUMMARY

Although surgical evacuation remains the treatment of choice for symptomatic cSDH, the appropriate treatment approach for asymptomatic patients is less clear. Initial medical treatment has focused on preventing further bleeding (with antithrombotic medication reversal strategies), and treating seizures regardless of the patient's clinical grade. However, the role of prophylactic seizure medication use is more controversial and is left to the discretion of the provider based on the patient's seizure risk.

Further investigation into the natural course of asymptomatic, small cSDH is necessary, along with the role of nonoperative alternatives for management. Early studies have shown potential for using medical therapies, as discussed here, either exclusively or as adjuncts to surgery, and this may prove to be more beneficial than previous watch-and-wait strategies. Future studies may show that, in certain cases, the necessity for surgical intervention may be avoided.

REFERENCES

1. Kolias AG, Chari A, Santarius T, et al. Chronic subdural haematoma: modern management and emerging therapies. Nat Rev Neurol 2014;10: 570–8.
2. Amirjamshidi A, Abouzari M, Rashidi A. Glasgow Coma Scale on admission is correlated with postoperative Glasgow Outcome Scale in chronic subdural hematoma. J Clin Neurosci 2007;14:1240–1.
3. Berghauser Pont LME, Dammers R, Schouten JW, et al. Clinical factors associated with outcome in chronic subdural hematoma: a retrospective cohort study of patients on preoperative corticosteroid therapy. Neurosurgery 2012;70:873–80 [discussion: 880].
4. Markwalder TM, Steinsiepe KF, Rohner M, et al. The course of chronic subdural hematomas after burr-hole craniostomy and closed-system drainage. J Neurosurg 1981;55:390–6.
5. Weigel R, Schmiedek P, Krauss JK. Outcome of contemporary surgery for chronic subdural haematoma: evidence based review. J Neurol Neurosurg Psychiatry 2003;74:937–43.
6. Taussky P, Hidalgo ET, Landolt H, et al. Age and salvageability: analysis of outcome of patients older than 65 years undergoing craniotomy for acute traumatic subdural hematoma. World Neurosurg 2012; 78:306–11.
7. Miranda LB, Braxton E, Hobbs J, et al. Chronic subdural hematoma in the elderly: not a benign disease. J Neurosurg 2011;114:72–6.
8. Ohno K, Maehara T, Ichimura K, et al. Low incidence of seizures in patients with chronic subdural haematoma. J Neurol Neurosurg Psychiatry 1993; 56:1231–3.
9. Grobelny BT, Ducruet AF, Zacharia BE, et al. Preoperative antiepileptic drug administration and the incidence of postoperative seizures following bur hole-treated chronic subdural hematoma. J Neurosurg 2009;111: 1257–62.

10. Rubin G, Rappaport ZH. Epilepsy in chronic subdural haematoma. Acta Neurochir (Wien) 1993; 123:39–42.

11. Sabo RA, Hanigan WC, Aldag JC. Chronic subdural hematomas and seizures: the role of prophylactic anticonvulsive medication. Surg Neurol 1995;43: 579–82.

12. Chen C-W, Kuo JR, Lin HJ, et al. Early postoperative seizures after burr-hole drainage for chronic subdural hematoma: correlation with brain CT findings. J Clin Neurosci 2004;11:706–9.

13. Radic JAE, Chou SH-Y, Du R, et al. Levetiracetam versus phenytoin: a comparison of efficacy of seizure prophylaxis and adverse event risk following acute or subacute subdural hematoma diagnosis. Neurocrit Care 2014;21:228–37.

14. Kruer RM, Harris LH, Goodwin H, et al. Changing trends in the use of seizure prophylaxis after traumatic brain injury: a shift from phenytoin to levetiracetam. J Crit Care 2013;28:883.e9-13.

15. Frati A, Salvati M, Mainiero F, et al. Inflammation markers and risk factors for recurrence in 35 patients with a posttraumatic chronic subdural hematoma: a prospective study. J Neurosurg 2004;100: 24–32.

16. Stanisic M, Aasen AO, Pripp AH, et al. Local and systemic pro-inflammatory and anti-inflammatory cytokine patterns in patients with chronic subdural hematoma: a prospective study. Inflamm Res 2012;61:845–52.

17. Kalamatianos T, Stavrinou LC, Koutsarnakis C, et al. PlGF and sVEGFR-1 in chronic subdural hematoma: implications for hematoma development. J Neurosurg 2013;118:353–7.

18. Sun TFD, Boet R, Poon WS. Non-surgical primary treatment of chronic subdural haematoma: Preliminary results of using dexamethasone. Br J Neurosurg 2005;19:327–33.

19. Delgado-López PD, Martín-Velasco V, Castilla-Díez JM, et al. Dexamethasone treatment in chronic subdural haematoma. Neurocirugia (Astur) 2009;20: 346–59.

20. Thotakura AK, Marabathina NR. Nonsurgical treatment of chronic subdural hematoma with steroids. World Neurosurg 2015;84:1968–72.

21. Prud'homme M, Mathieu F, Marcotte N, et al. A pilot placebo controlled randomized trial of dexamethasone for chronic subdural hematoma. Can J Neurol Sci 2016;43:284–90.

22. Dran G, Berthier F, Fontaine D, et al. Effectiveness of adjuvant corticosteroid therapy for chronic subdural hematoma: a retrospective study of 198 cases. Neurochirurgie 2007;53:477–82 [in French].

23. Cenic A, Bhandari M, Reddy K. Management of chronic subdural hematoma: a national survey and literature review. Can J Neurol Sci 2005;32:501–6.

24. Santarius T, Lawton R, Kirkpatrick PJ, et al. The management of primary chronic subdural haematoma: a questionnaire survey of practice in the United Kingdom and the Republic of Ireland. Br J Neurosurg 2008;22:529–34.

25. Berghauser Pont LME, Dippel DWJ, Verweij BH, et al. Ambivalence among neurologists and neurosurgeons on the treatment of chronic subdural hematoma: a national survey. Acta Neurol Belg 2013; 113:55–9.

26. Jain MK, Ridker PM. Anti-inflammatory effects of statins: clinical evidence and basic mechanisms. Nat Rev Drug Discov 2005;4:977–87.

27. Wang B, Sun L, Tian Y, et al. Effects of atorvastatin in the regulation of circulating EPCs and angiogenesis in traumatic brain injury in rats. J Neurol Sci 2012; 319:117–23.

28. Chen J, Zhang ZG, Li Y, et al. Statins induce angiogenesis, neurogenesis, and synaptogenesis after stroke. Ann Neurol 2003;53:743–51.

29. Kureishi Y, Luo Z, Shiojima I, et al. The HMG-CoA reductase inhibitor simvastatin activates the protein kinase Akt and promotes angiogenesis in normocholesterolemic animals. Nat Med 2000;6:1004–10.

30. Li T, Wang D, Tian Y, et al. Effects of atorvastatin on the inflammation regulation and elimination of subdural hematoma in rats. J Neurol Sci 2014;341: 88–96.

31. Weigel R, Hohenstein A, Schlickum L, et al. Angiotensin converting enzyme inhibition for arterial hypertension reduces the risk of recurrence in patients with chronic subdural hematoma possibly by an antiangiogenic mechanism. Neurosurgery 2007;61(4):788–92 [discussion: 792–3].

32. Neidert MC, Schmidt T, Mitova T, et al. Preoperative angiotensin converting enzyme inhibitor usage in patients with chronic subdural hematoma: Associations with initial presentation and clinical outcome. J Clin Neurosci 2016;28:82–6.

33. Poulsen FR, Munthe S, Søe M, et al. Perindopril and residual chronic subdural hematoma volumes six weeks after burr hole surgery: a randomized trial. Clin Neurol Neurosurg 2014;123:4–8.

34. Kageyama H, Toyooka T, Tsuzuki N, et al. Nonsurgical treatment of chronic subdural hematoma with tranexamic acid. J Neurosurg 2013;119:332–7.

Minimally Invasive Surgical Approaches for Chronic Subdural Hematomas

Ian A. Buchanan, MD, William J. Mack, MD*

KEYWORDS

- Chronic subdural hematoma • Burr hole • Twist drill • Craniostomy

KEY POINTS

- Chronic subdural hematomas have had an increasing incidence in modern neurosurgical practices because of the aging population.
- Twist drill craniostomy and burr hole craniostomy are the 2 minimally invasive approaches available for addressing chronic subdural hematomas. Of the two, burr hole craniostomy is the most widely used technique worldwide.
- Twist drill craniostomy is a relatively safe and effective first-line option for chronic subdural hematoma evacuation that obviates general anesthetic, making it an attractive option in high-risk cohorts.
- Reported estimates on cure rates, recurrence, morbidity, and mortality for the various treatment modalities are highly variable.
- Despite their prevalence, there is no consensus regarding first-line management for chronic subdural hematomas.

INTRODUCTION

Chronic subdural hematomas (cSDH) are one of the fastest growing neurologic conditions, fueled in part by an aging Western population and the bourgeoning use of anticoagulant and antiplatelet therapy.[1] In the United States alone, the total number of individuals 65 years and older is projected to double by the middle of this century, and, as a consequence, the disease burden from this clinical entity is expected to follow.[2] Current trends indicate that cSDHs are poised to become the most common intracranial diagnosis to require surgical intervention by year 2030, exceeding both primary brain tumors and metastases.[3,4] Given the substantial morbidity and mortality they carry, cSDHs therefore constitute a remarkable economic and social burden to societies worldwide.

CSDHs are the end product of liquefied blood degradation within the subdural space. Although trauma is often an inciting agent in their formation, roughly a third of patients have no such recollection, suggesting that even minor seemingly inconsequential events are precipitants of this pathologic condition.[5] The propensity for cSDH formation in the elderly can be explained by the shrinking brain volume within the confines of the cranial vault. As this occurs, tension on the bridging parasagittal veins that drain the cortical surface predisposes them to injury and hemorrhage at the dura-arachnoid interface. The theoretic subdural space, which is normally obliterated by tight adherence between the meningeal layers on account of dural border cells, is thus transformed by hematoma formation.[6]

Disclosure Statement: The authors have no commercial relationships or financial interests to disclose.
Department of Neurosurgery, Keck School of Medicine, University of Southern California, 1520 San Pablo Street, Suite 3800, Los Angeles, CA 90033, USA
* Corresponding author.
E-mail address: william.mack@med.usc.edu

neurosurgery.theclinics.com

Discovery of cSDHs in the elderly can be viewed as a harbinger of systemic pathologic conditions in much the same way that hip fractures are seen as a proxy for mortality. Recent studies suggest that the 1-year mortality rate in patients 70 years and older with newly diagnosed cSDH approaches 32%.[7] Besides age, other factors that predispose to cSDH formation include, but are not limited to, a history of trauma, hereditary bleeding diatheses, epilepsy, ethanol abuse, and anticoagulation. Of these, age and anticoagulant use have garnered the most attention in recent years for their contributions to increasing hematoma incidence. Anticoagulation increases the risk of cSDH by more than 40-fold relative to the general population.[8] Although the mechanism in this scenario may be the result of uncontrolled bleeding from a severed vessel, more common is that there is microbleeding that progresses unchecked from an asymptomatic hemorrhage to one with neurologic sequelae.[9]

Transformation of acute bleeding to chronic bleeding follows a series of pathologic processes in which there is fibrin deposition followed by subsequent organization, enzymatic fibrinolysis, and clot liquefaction.[2] In many cases, this process is sufficient to achieve complete resorption of the hematoma. However, in other instances, a chronic inflammatory reaction is set in motion, entailing dural border cell proliferation, collagen synthesis, and neomembrane formation with neovascularization. The latter is a seminal event in the formation of cSDHs, and this ingrowth of fragile capillaries into the neomembranes underlies their propensity for microhemorrhage with cyclical recurrence. Some even propose that antithrombotic and fibrinolytic substances are secreted by the neomembrane into the hematoma cavity, enabling persistence and gradual enlargement over time.[10,11]

Three primary techniques for addressing cSDH entail sequentially larger cranial openings for hematoma drainage: twist drill craniostomy (TDC), burr hole craniostomy (BHC), and craniotomy. The process of creating windows in the skull for intracranial conditions is not new but dates as far back as the Neolithic era (8000–5000 BC).[12] Trephination, or trepanation, represents the earliest attempt by prehistoric man at neurosurgery. Although its beginnings were likely mystical in origin and based on the magico-ritual practice of freeing evil spirits from within the skull, over time it evolved into a therapeutic process for depressed skull fractures and intracranial hematomas.[12] The earliest description is documented in the Hippocratic treatise, On Injuries of the Head, in which for the first time a systematic account is provided complete with indications, timing, and technical notes. After Hippocrates' publication, trephination became widespread. It has undergone numerous iterations over the centuries, but it was not until the advent of antisepsis and improved anesthesia in the nineteenth century that the craniotomy became cemented into modernity.[13]

Despite the increasing number of cSDH cases diagnosed annually, there is no consensus for their general management. Definitive evidence regarding the superiority of one surgical modality over the other is lacking, and the decision to treat is therefore determined on an individual basis after consideration of the patient's clinical status, comorbidities, and radiologic appearance of the hematoma. Here, we discuss minimally invasive approaches for cSDH management (TDC and BHC) along with adjunctive therapies with the potential for influencing cure rates, recurrence, and other complications.

CLINICAL PRESENTATION AND INDICATIONS FOR SURGERY

A symptomatic subdural hematoma that is chronic in nature can present in a multitude of ways, earning it the nickname *great imitator*.[14] This hematoma can occur over a protracted period with isolated cognitive decline mimicking dementia or can present acutely in the context of focal neurologic deficits, as seen in stroke, or dramatically with coma and even death. Symptoms result from increased intracranial pressure or mass effect on crucial structures. However, because cSDHs tend to develop slowly and in the context of marked brain atrophy, they may not become clinically apparent until they are of a large enough size for which compensation by the cortex is no longer possible. Symptoms most commonly include headache, nausea, emesis, drowsiness, vertigo, seizures, mental deterioration, gait instability, and limb paresis. When symptoms are exceptionally vague, diagnosis can sometimes prove difficult, because there is often no history of a traumatic event to trigger routine cranial imaging. However, continued advances in radiology and the widespread availability of computed tomography scanners have contributed to an increase in cSDH diagnosis.

CSDH appears as a crescent-shaped lesion along the cerebral convexity on computed tomography (CT) imaging. It readily crosses cranial suture lines and is hypodense in appearance but can contain hyperdense regions coinciding with areas of calcification or membrane formation. Identification of dense membranes or significant loculation at the time of diagnosis is important because it may influence the pursuit of a larger craniotomy in favor of more minimally invasive approaches. The decision to evacuate a cSDH is determined by clinical presentation and the radiographic size and features of a hematoma. Surgical drainage is recommended for hematomas greater than 1 cm in diameter regardless of symptoms,[15] but this threshold is rather arbitrary and absolute volumetric size cutoffs do not exist. Asymptomatic lesions or those producing only mild symptoms can be observed in a monitored setting with medical management. The justification here is that these lesions can sometimes resolve spontaneously without further sequelae.[16] However, once focal deficits or marked changes in neurologic status become evident, the consensus is that surgical drainage should be pursued as long as there are no medical contraindications.

SURGICAL TECHNIQUE
Preoperative Considerations

After radiographic confirmation of a cSDH, patients are typically admitted for serial neurologic examinations in a carefully monitored setting. Those who may require drainage are given nothing by mouth, and a routine preoperative workup is initiated to ensure clearance for the operating room. During this period, vigilance is maintained for any signs of clinical deterioration that would warrant acceleration of a surgical timeline. As in all arenas of critical care, the "ABCs" take precedence, and any patient with a Glasgow Coma Score of 8 or lower should be intubated. Unlike in trauma, insertion of an external ventricular drain for poor GCS is not indicated and, in fact, should be avoided because drainage of cerebrospinal fluid can exacerbate the underlying cSDH by increasing retraction on draining veins, in much the same way that aggressive lowering of settings in implanted ventriculoperitoneal shunts can give rise to subdural collections. In the event of impending herniation, diuresis can be attempted as a desperate bridging therapy to surgery. However, in stable patients its use should be avoided because intravascular volume depletion severely limits brain expansion postoperatively and increases the chances of hematoma recurrence.

With the burgeoning use of anticoagulant therapy in our aging society, these medications are increasingly being implicated in cSDH hospital admissions. A thorough medical history and routine hematology and coagulation studies should therefore be performed to help identify any underlying coagulopathy as the etiology of hematoma formation. When coagulation abnormalities are discovered, it is imperative that they be preemptively addressed during the initial evaluation. If the coagulopathy is iatrogenic in origin, offending agents

should be promptly discontinued to minimize the risks of enlargement from acute hemorrhage into a chronic hematoma. Additionally, the effects of antiplatelet and anticoagulant therapy should be promptly reversed. If life-threatening hematoma progression is imminent, it is universally accepted that rapid reversal be initiated regardless of the indication for anticoagulation use, as cessation of intracranial bleeding takes precedence over the preexisting medical indication that necessitated its use to begin with.

Antiepileptic pharmacotherapy is an important perioperative adjunct to consider in cSDH management. Seizure rates in patients who undergo drainage are highly variable and range from 2% to 19%.[17,18] This rate increases markedly if cortical injury is present secondary to concomitant trauma at the time of hematoma formation or if neomembrane violation occurs during cSDH evacuation.[19] Several published studies in cSDH patients posit that antiepileptic drug (AED) prophylaxis incurs unnecessary morbidity without reducing seizure frequency, except in certain high-risk cohorts.[17,20] Such high-risk patients include those with a documented history of seizures, underlying traumatic brain injury, or alcoholism. On the other hand, others strongly advocate for general AED use around the operative period, citing significant reductions in seizure rates, albeit with no impact on discharge outcomes.[21–23] These seemingly contradictory reports contribute to inconsistent AED use in cSDH treatment.

Although it is certainly reasonable to administer AEDs during the perioperative period, their use can increase the risk of falling in the elderly.[24] Special consideration should therefore be given when administering AEDs in those 65 years and older, as the increased risk of recurrent hemorrhage from falling must be weighed against the morbidity of seizures in this population.

Twist Drill Craniostomy

Surgical evacuation remains the gold standard for treating cSDHs symptomatic from mass effect. There are 3 primary surgical interventions for addressing cSDH: minimally invasive approaches, twist drill and burr hole craniostomy, and formal craniotomy. Craniotomy makes use of a bone flap (usually >30 mm), which is replaced after surgery usually with some form of plating system. It is the most invasive of the listed options and will be addressed elsewhere. TDC, as the name implies, is a percutaneous technique that entails the use of a handheld twist drill for creating a single cranial opening less than 10 mm. It is typically performed under local anesthesia at the patient's bedside and may be used in conjunction with or without subdural drain insertion or closed suction drainage attached to an implanted transosseous bolt.

TDC was first described by Tabaddor and Shulmon in 1977 when they reported on its efficacy as an alternative to larger craniotomies.[25] In the original description, a 1-cm incision is made over the hematoma. A craniostomy is then performed by placing a twist drill angled about 45° to the surface of the skull to avoid inadvertent injury to the underlying parenchyma. The dura and outer cSDH membrane can be violated with the drill but preferably with the use of a sharp needle in a more controlled fashion. A cannula is then directed into the longitudinal aspect of the hematoma and connected to a gravity drainage bag for ongoing evacuation of the subdural space. Since its development, TDC has been repeatedly validated as a first-line therapy in high-risk cohorts.[26,27] Its use is considered favorable in scenarios in which multiple comorbidities confer an unacceptably high risk for undergoing general anesthesia. One of its main disadvantages, however, is the increased risk for infection when performed bedside.

Several modifications have been made over the years to enhance the safety and sterility of TDC. In one such technique, a hollow screw or bolt is threaded down the craniostomy opening to set up a hermetically sealed drainage system, sometimes referred to as the subdural evacuating port system.[28,29] This modification not only minimizes infection, but obviates blind passage of a drain into the subdural space by relying on slight negative pressure for subdural evacuation and, hence, limits cortical injury. In another TDC variation, a special bolt is placed over the parietal eminence to facilitate instillation of oxygen or some other insufflation agent as the driving force for hematoma removal.[30] Often cited advantages of this technique include decreased likelihood for postoperative pneumocephalus and headache. Preliminary evidence suggests that these novel TDC modifications are at least equivalent, if not superior, in efficacy to their predecessor.[31]

Burr Hole Craniostomy

BHC is the most commonly used technique for evacuating cSDHs in many countries because of its low recurrence rate and low morbidity and mortality indices.[32–34] This technique was popularized by Markwalder and colleagues[35] in the 1980s after their report on its use as a viable first-line alternative to formal craniotomy. BHC can be performed under local anesthesia, but patients are typically taken to the operating room where they are placed under general or at least systemic anesthesia.

BHC consists of making 2 small cranial openings 10 to 30 mm in size along the cerebral convexity. These are made with the use of a high-speed drill and spaced some distance apart to facilitate saline irrigation between them. The dura is then opened and the leaflets bipolared to the edge of the craniostomy to ensure that the subdural space remains in communication with the cranial opening. Any subdural collection is then irrigated in a reciprocating fashion until the effluent becomes clear.

Although 2 burr holes are commonly used to allow for back-and-forth irrigation, a single burr hole may be used as well. There is no conclusive evidence specifying an optimal number of cranial openings, but there are data to suggest that use of a single craniostomy results in longer hospital stays and higher rates of recurrence and wound infection.[36] Alternatively, there is also evidence in the other direction suggesting that the number of holes has no influence whatsoever on outcomes.[37–39] Although it seems obvious that visualization of the effluent during reciprocating irrigation via a 2-hole technique provides visual feedback on the adequacy of cSDH evacuation and would therefore dictate its use, the number of craniostomies made remains entirely based on surgeon preference.

Current level I evidence is in strong support of closed-system drainage of the subdural space after burr holes because of significant reductions in recurrence and length of hospitalization and concomitant improvements in mortality.[40] A temporary subdural or subgaleal drain should therefore be left in place whenever feasible to evacuate any fluid that reaccumulates in the immediate postoperative period. Because subdural drain insertion carries a risk of cortical injury, epilepsy, and infection, subgaleal or subperiosteal drainage has been proposed as a less-invasive alternative. Preliminary studies show statistically equivalent recurrence and complication rates between the 2 approaches.[41–44] Further, prospective randomized trials are needed to sufficiently determine whether subgaleal and subdural drainage are indeed comparable in efficacy and outcome.

POSTOPERATIVE CONSIDERATIONS

After treatment, strict blood pressure control within the normotensive range is paramount to minimizing acute hemorrhage in the postoperative period. An immediate postoperative CT scan should be obtained to assess the adequacy of drainage and establish a baseline for comparison going forward. If the residual clot burden is minimal and the patient found to be at their neurologic baseline, diet can be advanced by postoperative day 1. Use of perioperative antibiotics for gram-positive skin flora is generally not required beyond the first 24 hours. As the rates of recurrence are not negligible, patients should be carefully monitored for signs of reaccumulation resulting in new neurologic deficit. In otherwise asymptomatic patients, CT imaging should be repeated 1 to 2 weeks after surgery to screen for hematoma recurrence.

Early postoperative mobilization whenever feasible is one of the basic tenets of surgical management. This is especially important in the frail and elderly who are predisposed to pneumonia, deep venous thrombosis, and pulmonary emboli, well-known complications of prolonged immobilization. Notwithstanding the benefits of early mobilization, there is some evidence to suggest that bed rest promotes brain expansion and thus reduces cSDH recurrence.[45,46] This practice is however highly controversial, and only about 50% of surgeons subscribe to its use.[32,34] Randomized, controlled trials have been conducted to assess the relative contributions of postoperative position on hematoma recurrence and have reached differing conclusions. Work by Nakajima and colleagues[47] found that patient posture had no significant impact on the likelihood of cSDH recurrence. This finding has been confirmed by other studies but with an increased tendency toward medical complications—pneumonia and urinary tract infections—in the immobilized group.[48] Conversely, Abouzari and colleagues[45] discovered that patients who had the head of their bed elevated by 30° to 40° immediately after evacuation had significantly higher rates of hematoma re-formation relative to those maintained in a recumbent position. Because both studies were severely limited by the small size of their cohorts, additional work is needed before any conclusive guidelines can be established on this aspect of cSDH management.

All cSDH patients should have sequential compression devices applied at the time of admission, provided there are no contraindications. Postoperatively, anyone with impaired mobility should be started on thromboembolism prophylaxis with low-dose unfractionated heparin or its low-molecular-weight variant as soon as it is deemed safe by the operating provider. In the case of adequate intraoperative hemostasis, this could be in as little as 12 to 24 hours after surgery but preferably after removal of any drainage catheters. One obvious caveat of prophylaxis initiation is the potential for increases in hematoma recurrence. In one retrospective study, these rates were reported to be as high as 2-fold for enoxaparin.[49] Evidence-based guidelines of the optimal timing for introducing deep vein thrombosis chemoprophylaxis are lacking, and the decision is therefore at the discretion of the treating physician and may be guided by neuroimaging.

For those at high risk for thromboembolic events (eg, mechanical cardiac valves), conversion to full-dose anticoagulation is a different matter altogether and relies on a delicate balance of the likelihood of hematoma recurrence against the risk of thrombotic complications while off pharmacotherapy. To that effect, rather than a fixed interval to resumption, the neurosurgeon must assess every case individually to determine the optimal cessation period based on intraoperative findings and whether postoperative imaging demonstrates acute hemorrhage or signs of hematoma recurrence. Other important factors to consider include functional status, comorbidities, indication for anticoagulation, and likelihood for further falls or head trauma. Empirical evidence is sparse, but some data indicate that warfarin can be reintroduced safely within 72 hours of operation in the most high risk of cohorts.[50,51] There is also a dearth of information on the timing for reinitiating antiplatelet agents; however, some data suggest that this can be done safely within 7 days of any interventions.[52] Regardless of the length of time that full-dose anticoagulation or antiplatelet therapy was withheld, it would be prudent to obtain follow-up imaging after a therapeutic dose has been reinstituted and the patient proven to be within the desired therapeutic range.

SURGICAL COMPLICATIONS AND MANAGEMENT

Barring catastrophic circumstances, the most worrisome complication in the management of cSDH is a recurrence that warrants repeat surgery. Reported recurrence rates in the literature are highly variable and range anywhere from 0% to 33% for BHCs and TDCs.[2,5,53,54] However, those requiring reoperation only account for about 10% to 20%. Although the etiology for re-accumulation can be multifactorial, the most likely culprit is failure of brain expansion to eliminate intracranial dead space. This failure is more common in scenarios in which the original hematoma contained complex features not amenable to drainage by minimally invasive techniques (eg, solid clot or multiple membranes with loculation).[55] Known risk factors besides poor brain re-expansion and loculated membranes include age, large original hematoma size, bilateral lesions,[56,57] cerebral atrophy, anticoagulant or antiplatelet use, alcoholism,[58] presence of cerebrospinal fluid shunt,[59] pneumocephalus,[60] and persistent postoperative of midline shift.[61] Irrespective of the causal pathologic conditions, repeat surgical drainage via the original methodology is efficacious in more than 70% of cases, although formal craniotomy for maximal exposure would certainly be reasonable.[62]

Several strategies have been developed over the years to lessen cSDH recurrence by encouraging brain expansion and obliterating dead space. Avoidance of diuresis around the time of surgery, prompt intravenous return of perioperative fluid losses, and gentle hyperhydration are all practices devised with such reasoning in mind.[63] In a like manner, high-flow oxygen supplementation via nonrebreather mask and prolonged bed rest with recumbency were instituted to minimize pneumocephalus as a nidus for hematoma reformation. Despite these efforts, the only proven method for decreasing the possibility of relapse is intraoperative placement of a closed-system catheter for draining the subdural space. Initial trials validating the practice were all conducted with subdural drains, but early results on subgaleal catheters seem just as promising.[2,43]

The elderly are particularly susceptible to even minor complications from general anesthesia. These can blossom into adverse events that lead to prolonged ventilator dependence, untimely tracheostomy with gastrostomy, and even death. It is therefore crucial that vigilance be maintained over the course of their hospitalization so that ostensibly trivial matters can be addressed in a timely manner. These and other common complications encountered in cSDH management are summarized in **Table 1**.

SURGICAL OUTCOMES

Surgical evacuation remains the gold standard for treating patients symptomatic from a radiologically confirmed cSDH. Drainage facilitates prompt reversal of neurologic deficits and results in a favorable outcome in most patients.[2,64] With the advent of better health care, patients are living well beyond their anticipated life expectancies, and studies show surgical treatment to be safe and efficacious even in the eldest of elderly, including nonagenarians and centenarians.[64] Three principal surgical modalities exist and they use progressively larger cranial openings to address the underlying hematoma. Although the treatment algorithm is guided by the radiographic features of the cSDH, most lesions without calcification or extensive membranes can be addressed via any of the 3 modalities. There is no class I evidence available directly comparing techniques and, as a consequence, the optimal modality remains controversial with the final decision often being determined by surgeon preference.

Much of the comparison across techniques can be found in various comprehensive systematic reviews and meta-analyses.[2,62,63,65] In a 2003 review, Weigel and colleagues[62] determined that TDC, BHC, and craniotomy had similar cure and mortality rates. However, formal craniotomy was found to have a substantially higher morbidity profile (12.3%) when compared with minimally invasive approaches, such as TDC (3%; $P<.001$) and BHC (3.8%; $P<.001$). Interestingly, when recurrence rates were tallied, TDC (33%) proved far less effective at preventing relapses relative to BHC (12%; $P<.001$) and craniotomy (10.8%). This finding led to their support for BHC as the preferred first-line approach in light of its favorable cure-to-complication ratio.

A subsequent meta-analysis by Ducruet and colleagues[2] similarly found that TDC had the highest rates of recurrence (28.1%) versus BHC (11.7%, $P<.0001$) and craniotomy (19.4%, $P<.0001$). However, unlike the aforementioned study, it was BHC that carried significantly higher complication rates (9.3%) compared with TDC (2.5%; $P<.001$) and craniotomy (3.9%; $P = .0046$). Because TDC had a disproportionately larger number of patients who showed neurologic improvement, the authors advocated for its use over its counterparts, particularly when the cost implications of avoiding a trip to the operating room were considered. The challenge with distilling recommendations from these comparative data is that much of the analyses are based on studies with unclear or high risks of bias. It is not surprising then that more recent meta-analyses failed to highlight the superiority of one technique over the other, citing no significant differences regarding cure rates, recurrence, morbidity, or mortality.[63,65] Carefully designed,

Table 1
Procedure-specific and medical complications associated with chronic subdural hematoma management

Surgical Complications	Medical Complications
• Cortical injury	• Ischemic stroke
• Intracerebral hemorrhage	• Myocardial infarction
• Seizure	• Hospital-acquired respiratory infection
• Status epilepticus	• Ventilator dependence requiring tracheostomy/gastrostomy
• Surgical site infection	
• Subdural empyema	• Venous thrombosis
• Tension pneumocephalus	• Pulmonary embolism
	• Urinary tract infection

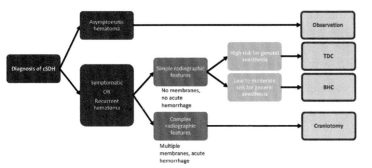

Fig. 1. Potential decision matrix for determining the appropriate surgical intervention for cSDHs.

prospective, randomized trials are needed to further elucidate the optimal method of chronic SDH evacuation.

Because evidence-based guidelines are lacking, the question of which technique to use must therefore be answered by the clinical status of the patient and the radiographic appearance of the hematoma (**Fig. 1**). Acute hemorrhage or the presence of multiloculated, thickened or calcified membranes calls for a larger craniotomy than is offered by minimally invasive techniques. In the absence of complex features, TDC and BHC are the first line of surgical therapy, with BHC being the preferred method based on its favorable cure-to-complication profile. However, in high-risk surgical cohorts TDC is favored for its bedside application and circumvention of general anesthesia. Regardless of the minimally invasive strategy used, postoperative drain placement is now the standard of care based on statistically significant reductions in recurrence and hospital length of stay.[40]

REFERENCES

1. Kolias AG, Chari A, Santarius T, et al. Chronic subdural haematoma: modern management and emerging therapies. Nat Rev Neurol 2014;10(10):570–8.

2. Ducruet AF, Grobelny BT, Zacharia BE, et al. The surgical management of chronic subdural hematoma. Neurosurg Rev 2012;35(2):155–69 [discussion: 169].

3. Filippini G. Epidemiology of primary central nervous system tumors. Handb Clin Neurol 2012;104:3–22.

4. Gavrilovic IT, Posner JB. Brain metastases: epidemiology and pathophysiology. J Neurooncol 2005; 75(1):5–14.

5. Gelabert-Gonzalez M, Iglesias-Pais M, García-Allut A, et al. Chronic subdural haematoma: surgical treatment and outcome in 1000 cases. Clin Neurol Neurosurg 2005;107(3):223–9.

6. Haines DE, Harkey HL, al-Mefty O. The "subdural" space: a new look at an outdated concept. Neurosurgery 1993;32(1):111–20.

7. Miranda LB, Braxton E, Hobbs J, et al. Chronic subdural hematoma in the elderly: not a benign disease. J Neurosurg 2011;114(1):72–6.

8. Rust T, Kiemer N, Erasmus A. Chronic subdural haematomas and anticoagulation or anti-thrombotic therapy. J Clin Neurosci 2006;13(8):823–7.

9. Roob G, Schmidt R, Kapeller P, et al. MRI evidence of past cerebral microbleeds in a healthy elderly population. Neurology 1999;52(5):991–4.

10. Ito H, Yamamoto S, Komai T, et al. Role of local hyperfibrinolysis in the etiology of chronic subdural hematoma. J Neurosurg 1976;45(1):26–31.

11. Ito H, Komai T, Yamamoto S. Fibrinolytic enzyme in the lining walls of chronic subdural hematoma. J Neurosurg 1978;48(2):197–200.

12. Newman WC, Chivukula S, Grandhi R. From mystics to modern times: a history of craniotomy & religion. World Neurosurg 2016;92:148–50.

13. Finger S, Clower WT. Victor Horsley on "trephining in pre-historic times". Neurosurgery 2001;48(4):911–7 [discussion: 917–8].

14. Potter JF, Fruin AH. Chronic subdural hematoma–the "great imitator". Geriatrics 1977;32(6):61–6.

15. Greenberg M. Chronic subdural hematoma. Handbook of Neurosurgery. 7th edition. New York: Thieme; 2010.

16. Parlato C, Guarracino A, Moraci A. Spontaneous resolution of chronic subdural hematoma. Surg Neurol 2000;53(4):312–5 [discussion: 315–7].

17. Ohno K, Maehara T, Ichimura K, et al. Low incidence of seizures in patients with chronic subdural haematoma. J Neurol Neurosurg Psychiatry 1993;56(11):1231–3.

18. Ratilal BO, Pappamikail L, Costa J, et al. Anticonvulsants for preventing seizures in patients with chronic subdural haematoma. Cochrane Database Syst Rev 2013;(6):CD004893.

19. Temkin NR. Risk factors for posttraumatic seizures in adults. Epilepsia 2003;44(Suppl 10):18–20.

20. Rubin G, Rappaport ZH. Epilepsy in chronic subdural haematoma. Acta Neurochir (Wien) 1993; 123(1–2):39–42.

21. Sabo RA, Hanigan WC, Aldag JC. Chronic subdural hematomas and seizures: the role of prophylactic anticonvulsive medication. Surg Neurol 1995;43(6): 579–82.

22. Grobelny BT, Ducruet AF, Zacharia BE, et al. Preoperative antiepileptic drug administration and the incidence of postoperative seizures following bur hole-treated chronic subdural hematoma. J Neurosurg 2009;111(6):1257–62.

23. Chen CW, Kuo JR, Lin HJ, et al. Early post-operative seizures after burr-hole drainage for chronic subdural hematoma: correlation with brain CT findings. J Clin Neurosci 2004;11(7):706–9.

24. Ferreri S, Roth MT, Casteel C, et al. Methodology of an ongoing, randomized controlled trial to prevent falls through enhanced pharmaceutical care. Am J Geriatr Pharmacother 2008;6(2):61–81.

25. Tabaddor K, Shulmon K. Definitive treatment of chronic subdural hematoma by twist-drill craniostomy and closed-system drainage. J Neurosurg 1977;46(2):220–6.

26. Hubschmann OR. Twist drill craniostomy in the treatment of chronic and subacute subdural hematomas in severely ill and elderly patients. Neurosurgery 1980;6(3):233–6.

27. Ramnarayan R, Arulmurugan B, Wilson PM, et al. Twist drill craniostomy with closed drainage for chronic subdural haematoma in the elderly: an effective method. Clin Neurol Neurosurg 2008; 110(8):774–8.

28. Emonds N, Hassler WE. New device to treat chronic subdural hematoma–hollow screw. Neurol Res 1999; 21(1):77–8.

29. Rughani AI, Lin C, Dumont TM, et al. A case-comparison study of the subdural evacuating port system in treating chronic subdural hematomas. J Neurosurg 2010;113(3):609–14.

30. Takeda N, Sasaki K, Oikawa A, et al. A new simple therapeutic method for chronic subdural hematoma without irrigation and drainage. Acta Neurochir (Wien) 2006;148(5):541–6.

31. Kubo S, Takimoto H, Nakata H, et al. Carbon dioxide insufflation for chronic subdural haematoma: a simple addition to burr-hole irrigation and closed-system drainage. Br J Neurosurg 2003;17(6): 547–50.

32. Cenic A, Bhandari M, Reddy K. Management of chronic subdural hematoma: a national survey and literature review. Can J Neurol Sci 2005;32(4):501–6.

33. Nayil K, Ramzan A, Sajad A, et al. Subdural hematomas: an analysis of 1181 Kashmiri patients. World Neurosurg 2012;77(1):103–10.

34. Santarius T, Lawton R, Kirkpatrick PJ, et al. The management of primary chronic subdural haematoma: a questionnaire survey of practice in the United Kingdom and the Republic of Ireland. Br J Neurosurg 2008;22(4):529–34.

35. Markwalder TM, Steinsiepe KF, Rohner M, et al. The course of chronic subdural hematomas after burr-hole craniostomy and closed-system drainage. J Neurosurg 1981;55(3):390–6.

36. Taussky P, Fandino J, Landolt H. Number of burr holes as independent predictor of postoperative recurrence in chronic subdural haematoma. Br J Neurosurg 2008;22(2):279–82.

37. Kansal R, Nadkarni T, Goel A. Single versus double burr hole drainage of chronic subdural hematomas. A study of 267 cases. J Clin Neurosci 2010;17(4): 428–9.

38. Han HJ, Park CW, Kim EY, et al. One vs. Two Burr Hole Craniostomy in Surgical Treatment of Chronic Subdural Hematoma. J Korean Neurosurg Soc 2009;46(2):87–92.

39. Belkhair S, Pickett G. One versus double burr holes for treating chronic subdural hematoma meta-analysis. Can J Neurol Sci 2013;40(1):56–60.

40. Santarius T, Kirkpatrick PJ, Ganesan D, et al. Use of drains versus no drains after burr-hole evacuation of chronic subdural haematoma: a randomised controlled trial. Lancet 2009;374(9695):1067–73.

41. Gazzeri R, Galarza M, Neroni M, et al. Continuous subgaleal suction drainage for the treatment of chronic subdural haematoma. Acta Neurochir (Wien) 2007;149(5):487–93 [discussion: 493].

42. Zumofen D, Regli L, Levivier M, et al. Chronic subdural hematomas treated by burr hole trepanation and a subperiosteal drainage system. Neurosurgery 2009;64(6):1116–21 [discussion: 1121–2].

43. Bellut D, Woernle CM, Burkhardt JK, et al. Subdural drainage versus subperiosteal drainage in burr-hole trepanation for symptomatic chronic subdural hematomas. World Neurosurg 2012;77(1):111–8.

44. Kaliaperumal C, Khalil A, Fenton E, et al. A prospective randomised study to compare the utility and outcomes of subdural and subperiosteal drains for the treatment of chronic subdural haematoma. Acta Neurochir (Wien) 2012;154(11):2083–8 [discussion : 2088–9].

45. Abouzari M, Rashidi A, Rezaii J, et al. The role of postoperative patient posture in the recurrence of traumatic chronic subdural hematoma after burr-hole surgery. Neurosurgery 2007;61(4):794–7 [discussion: 797].

46. Choudhury AR. Avoidable factors that contribute to complications in the surgical treatment of chronic subdural haematoma. Acta Neurochir (Wien) 1994; 129(1–2):15–9.

47. Nakajima H, Yasui T, Nishikawa M, et al. The role of postoperative patient posture in the recurrence of chronic subdural hematoma: a prospective randomized trial. Surg Neurol 2002;58(6):385–7 [discussion: 387].

48. Kurabe S, Ozawa T, Watanabe T, et al. Efficacy and safety of postoperative early mobilization for chronic subdural hematoma in elderly patients. Acta Neurochir (Wien) 2010;152(7):1171–4.

49. Tahsim-Oglou Y, Beseoglu K, Hänggi D, et al. Factors predicting recurrence of chronic subdural

haematoma: the influence of intraoperative irrigation and low-molecular-weight heparin thromboprophylaxis. Acta Neurochir (Wien) 2012;154(6):1063–7 [discussion: 1068].

50. Yeon JY, Kong DS, Hong SC. Safety of early warfarin resumption following burr hole drainage for warfarin-associated subacute or chronic subdural hemorrhage. J Neurotrauma 2012;29(7):1334–41.

51. Kawamata T, Takeshita M, Kubo O, et al. Management of intracranial hemorrhage associated with anticoagulant therapy. Surg Neurol 1995;44(5): 438–42 [discussion: 443].

52. Torihashi K, Sadamasa N, Yoshida K, et al. Independent predictors for recurrence of chronic subdural hematoma: a review of 343 consecutive surgical cases. Neurosurgery 2008;63(6):1125–9 [discussion: 1129].

53. Ohba S, Kinoshita Y, Nakagawa T, et al. The risk factors for recurrence of chronic subdural hematoma. Neurosurg Rev 2013;36(1):145–9 [discussion: 149–50].

54. Baechli H, Nordmann A, Bucher HC, et al. Demographics and prevalent risk factors of chronic subdural haematoma: results of a large single-center cohort study. Neurosurg Rev 2004;27(4):263–6.

55. Ramachandran R, Hegde T. Chronic subdural hematomas–causes of morbidity and mortality. Surg Neurol 2007;67(4):367–72 [discussion: 372–3].

56. Kung WM, Hung KS, Chiu WT, et al. Quantitative assessment of impaired postevacuation brain re-expansion in bilateral chronic subdural haematoma: possible mechanism of the higher recurrence rate. Injury 2012;43(5):598–602.

57. Tugcu B, Tanriverdi O, Baydin S, et al. Can recurrence of chronic subdural hematoma be predicted? A retrospective analysis of 292 cases. J Neurol Surg A Cent Eur Neurosurg 2014;75(1):37–41.

58. Sonne NM, Tonnesen H. The influence of alcoholism on outcome after evacuation of subdural haematoma. Br J Neurosurg 1992;6(2):125–30.

59. Delgado PD, Cogolludo FJ, Mateo O, et al. Early prognosis in chronic subdural hematomas. Multivariate analysis of 137 cases. Rev Neurol 2000;30(9): 811–7 [in Spanish].

60. Mori K, Maeda M. Surgical treatment of chronic subdural hematoma in 500 consecutive cases: clinical characteristics, surgical outcome, complications, and recurrence rate. Neurol Med Chir (Tokyo) 2001;41(8):371–81.

61. Chon KH, Lee JM, Koh EJ, et al. Independent predictors for recurrence of chronic subdural hematoma. Acta Neurochir (Wien) 2012;154(9): 1541–8.

62. Weigel R, Schmiedek P, Krauss JK. Outcome of contemporary surgery for chronic subdural haematoma: evidence based review. J Neurol Neurosurg Psychiatry 2003;74(7):937–43.

63. Ivamoto HS, Lemos HP Jr, Atallah AN. Surgical treatments for chronic subdural hematomas: a comprehensive systematic review. World Neurosurg 2016; 86:399–418.

64. Lee L, Ker J, Ng HY, et al. Outcomes of chronic subdural hematoma drainage in nonagenarians and centenarians: a multicenter study. J Neurosurg 2016;124(2):546–51.

65. Almenawer SA, Farrokhyar F, Hong C, et al. Chronic subdural hematoma management: a systematic review and meta-analysis of 34,829 patients. Ann Surg 2014;259(3):449–57.

Craniotomy for Treatment of Chronic Subdural Hematoma

Isaac Josh Abecassis, MD[a],*, Louis J. Kim, MD[a,b]

KEYWORDS

- Chronic subdural hematoma • Craniotomy • Burr hole craniostomy

KEY POINTS

- Surgical intervention for chronic subdural hematomas (cSDHs) should be considered in cases of failed medical/conservative management or radiographic progression or with evidence of neurologic symptoms or deficit.
- Burr hole craniostomy (BHC) remains the gold standard for initially approaching cSDH, especially if liquefied and nonseptated.
- Craniotomy is particularly useful in treating cSDHs in cases of recurrence or with radiographic evidence of membranes.
- Craniotomy is associated with a higher morbidity and mortality than BHC and twist drill craniostomy (TDC), although with a lower complication rate than BHC and rates of recurrence similar to TDC.
- There is no reliably proved advantage to performing an aggressive total membranectomy.

INTRODUCTION

cSDHs are one of the more commonly encountered pathologies in neurologic surgery, with an estimated incidence of 1 to 2 in 100,000, a predilection for the elderly with a male predominance,[1,2] and a predicted rise in incidence secondary to increasing life expectancy in developed countries. Risk factors include a history of trauma, alcohol abuse, seizures, the presence of cerebrospinal fluid diversion (eg, ventriculoperitoneal shunt), and coagulopathies or anticoagulation. The underlying pathophysiology likely relates to an inflammatory process in the dura mater and subdural space in response to acute hemorrhage or some other insult. Subsequent neovascularization, formation of macrocapillaries, and vascular hyperpermeability lead to exudation and can contribute to hematoma enlargement, and higher rates of exudation have been correlated with worse clinical status.[3] The major culprit behind hematoma enlargement, however, remains the microhemorrhages associated with rupture of the fragile vessels generated with neovascularization. The natural history of cSDH depends largely on patient-specific conditions, although spontaneous resolution is possible.[4] Clinical severity of cSDH can be quantified with the Markwalder grading system[5] (**Table 1**). Radiographically, cSDH can be categorized into 1 of 5 categories based on CT imaging characteristics, as proposed in the Nomura classification system,[6] including (1) high density, (2) isodensity, (3) low density, (4) mixed density, and (5) layering lesions. Primary management for a symptomatic lesion is usually with surgical intervention, via (1) TDC – which can be done under local anesthetic in cases of medically complex patients, (2) BHC, or (3) craniotomy bone flap

Disclosure Statement: The authors have nothing to disclose.
[a] Department of Neurological Surgery, Harborview Medical Center, University of Washington, 325 9th Avenue, Box 359924, Seattle, WA 98104, USA; [b] Department of Radiology, Harborview Medical Center, University of Washington, 325 9th Avenue, 1st floor, 1 West Hospital, Seattle, WA 98104, USA
* Corresponding author.
E-mail address: abecassi@u.washington.edu

Neurosurg Clin N Am 28 (2017) 229–237
http://dx.doi.org/10.1016/j.nec.2016.11.005
1042-3680/17/© 2016 Elsevier Inc. All rights reserved.

Table 1
Markwalder scale for grading clinical condition in chronic subdural hematoma

Grade 0	No neurologic deficits
Grade 1	Mild symptoms (ie, headache, absent or mild neurologic deficits like reflex asymmetry)
Grade 2	Drowsiness or disoriented with variable neurologic deficit (ie, hemiparesis)
Grade 3	Stupor, severe focal neurologic deficit (ie, hemiplegia)
Grade 4	Coma, posturing, or absence of motor response to noxious stimulation

From Markwalder TM, Steinsiepe KF, Rohner M, et al. The course of chronic subdural hematomas after burr-hole craniostomy and closed-system drainage. J Neurosurg 1981;55(3):390–6; with permission.

(ie, >30 mm), although medical use of dexamethasone in some patients is a viable option used in international case series with comparable clinical outcomes.[7] There are several variations with craniotomy that are used, including a minicraniotomy (usually defined as 30–40 mm diameter), minicraniectomy, and either partial or full membranectomy. The goal of this article is to discuss the role of craniotomy in treating cSDH.

METHODS

The authors systematically reviewed the literature, using PubMed, with the search terms "chronic subdural hematoma", "craniotomy", and "outcomes". Any studies with only TDC or BHC as a surgical intervention or articles that combined outcomes of craniotomy with another subgroup were excluded. Non-English articles were also excluded. Patient cohort details, mortality, clinical outcomes, recurrence rate, and complication rates were documented for each study. Risk factors for either "poor" clinical outcomes or recurrence requiring operative intervention were documented as well as each group's specific definition of "poor outcome." Finally, the authors' institutional philosophy for triage of cSDH, surgical design, patient selection, and details of operation for performing a craniotomy were reviewed.

INDICATIONS/CONTRAINDICATIONS

Indications for craniotomy include any sort of symptomatic clot or fluid collection (ie, focal neurologic deficit related to the clot), with or without

failed conservative or less invasive (ie, BHC) management. Possible symptoms include headache, nausea or vomiting, seizures (either focally related to clot or generalized), weakness or numbness contralateral to the lesion, and aphasia for lesions on the dominant hemisphere. Evidence of the radiographic progression during a course of conservative observation is also a reasonable indication for consideration of operative intervention.

The selection of surgical technique is a topic of debate[8] and unfortunately largely understudied; a recent systematic review published by Ivamoto and colleagues[9] identified 24 randomized controlled trials (RCTs) in the surgical management of cSDHs, including comparisons, such as using a subdural drain postoperatively or using 1 versus 2 burr holes. The only RCT associated with craniotomy compared it to medical management with mannitol, and the trial was aborted after the first 7 patients in the medical arm had to cross over to the surgical arm.[10] It is generally a reasonable strategy to approach cSDH with BHC initially, because this procedure seems to achieve an ideal balance of limiting complications, mortality, and recurrence compared with TDC and craniotomy.[11] Still, surgeons should consider craniotomy in cases of (1) recurrence despite prior surgical intervention or (2) clots with evidence of membranes, which might inhibit evacuation via burr holes. Some investigators argue for performing contrasted MRI preoperatively, because this can highlight membranes and define particular cases where craniotomy may be useful as an upfront modality.[12–14] **Fig. 1** depicts a theoretical example of different membrane organization and triage strategy; in a study by Tanikawa and colleagues,27 patients with "type C" membranes (ie, extensive and multilayered on T2 MRI) treated with BHC had longer hospital stays, higher re-operation rates, and worse neurological outcomes compared to those treated with craniotomy. **Fig. 2** demonstrates an example of a mixed subacute/chronic SDH approached with craniotomy as an initial strategy given radiographic evidence of significant membranes.

SURGICAL TECHNIQUE
Preoperative Planning

Preoperatively, patients with either frank seizures or clinical behavior suspicious for seizures (ie, intermittent weakness or aphasia) should be loaded and maintained on an antiepileptic drug (AED) regimen appropriate to seizure type, although if seizure symptomatology is mild, it is sometimes reasonable to give surgical intervention an opportunity for relieving seizures, in which

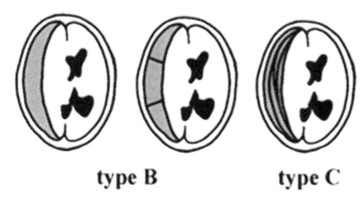

type B   type C

Fig. 1. Schema of intrahematomal structure as depicted by T2-weighted MRI. Left side of figure depicts a type B hematoma without any intrahematomal membrane. Middle of figure shows a type B hematoma with a monolayer multilobule hematoma. Right side of figure shows a type C hematoma, with a multilayer hematoma. (*From* Tanikawa M, Mase M, Yamada K, et al. Surgical treatment of chronic subdural hematoma based on intrahematomal membrane structure on MRI. Acta Neurochir (Wien) 2001;143:613–9; with permission.)

case AEDs can be avoided completely. If admitted through an emergency department, patients can be monitored on the normal wards (ie, infrequent neurochecks) with a nonemergent surgical plan unless there is significant mass effect, focal neurologic deficits, or severe symptoms. Emergent intervention should be considered in the event of new neurologic deficits, like weakness, because these can be permanent and due to vascular compression from mass effect. Basic preoperative laboratory tests should be obtained, and any coagulopathies should be corrected prior to surgical intervention. For patients on aspirin, the authors typically administer 1 U of platelets at the time of skin incision and plan to hold the medication anywhere from 48 hours to 2 weeks postoperatively, depending on the indication. The authors treat preoperative Coumadin/anticoagulation with fresh frozen plasma reversal and hold the medication in a similar time frame as for aspirin.

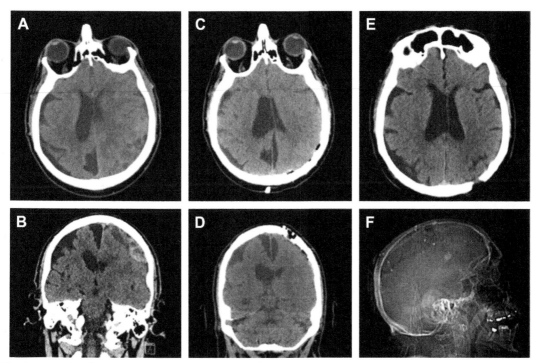

Fig. 2. Example of cSDH treated with craniotomy upfront. (*A,B*) Pre-operative head CT, demonstrating evidence of membranous subdural clot, mixed density, with local mass effect (axial and coronal cuts, respectively). (*C,D*) Post operative head CT demonstrating effective clot evacuation (axial and coronal cuts, respectively). (*E*) 6 week follow up head CT demonstrating persistent treatment (axial cut). (*F*) Lateral skull film demonstrating the extent of craniotomy.

In reviewing imaging, coronal reformats of head CT are particularly useful for planning craniotomy, especially in cases of minicraniotomy planned. Identification of the superior temporal line is useful to estimate cranial and caudal extension and extent of craniotomy in that plane, whereas identification of the clot in relation to the external auditory meatus helps to define the anterior and posterior boundaries.

Patient Positioning

Patients are positioned supine, with all pressure points padded appropriately and a shoulder bump under the ipsilateral side to promote exposure of the calvarium of the operative side. Either a horseshoe head-holder or Mayfield 3-point pin fixation can be used, although the authors' preference with any craniotomy is the latter. Attention is directed toward preoperative imaging to ensure that pins are not placed into the frontal sinus, and deliberate care is directed toward exposing a full calvarium for surgical preparation in the rare but potentially hazardous situation where conversion to a full-sized trauma-style craniotomy is necessary (ie, exposure of the zygomatic process, significant posterior extension into the occipital region, medial to the midline, and anterior up to the forehead). The head is slightly turned but without any kinking of the neck both for airway stability and to ensure proper venous drainage through the jugular veins. A curvilinear incision is planned along the theoretic blueprint of a trauma-style, reverse-question-mark incision. Alternatively, if a larger craniotomy is planned, a full or mini reverse-question-mark style incision can be planned.

Surgical Procedure

After exposing the calvarium, 1 or 2 burr holes are fashioned along the borders of the craniotomy. A Penfield #3 is used to strip the dura from the inner surface of bone prior to using the craniotome to fashion the craniotomy. Care should be taken to not extend the craniotomy over the superior sagittal sinus nor tear the dura along the medial border of the bony exposure to avoid cortical venous injury. Epidural tack-up stitches are placed with 4-0 neurolon stitches along the perimeter of the craniotomy. The dura is opened in a cruciate or stellate fashion. It is not necessary to identify the entire perimeter of the membrane/clot, because a full membranectomy is not essential. The outer layer of the membrane is entered and gently irrigated, because the boundaries are explored up until the perimeter of the craniotomy. Gentle irrigation of the inner, cortical membrane

layer can be performed, although aggressive traction and resection are not advised, because there can be adhesions to the cortical brain surface/veins, and these can cause new hemorrhage. All visible membrane (outer layer) is coagulated with bipolar cautery, including just under the edges of the craniotomy. When hemostasis is achieved, the bone flap is replaced with titanium plates and screws. The authors do not place any dural substitute over the cavity or close the dura tightly, because this promotes an outlet for subdural drainage via a subgaleal drain.

POTENTIAL COMPLICATIONS AND MANAGEMENT

Postoperative complications related to craniotomy for cSDH can be grouped into medical complications related to hospitalization and more surgically specific complications. Medical complications are more common than surgical ones, partially owing to older, medical complicated typical cSDH patients. Rates are intermittently reported in various series and include urinary tract infection, pneumonia, deep venous thrombosis with or without pulmonary embolus, myocardial infarction, pneumothorax, stroke, and so forth. Higher rates of complication seem to be associated with longer hospital stays and more extensive preoperative medical comorbidities, although formal validation in the cSDH population remains to be demonstrated. **Table 2** summarize the existing studies in the literature with craniotomy as compared to other treatment modalities for cSDH, with the various outcomes assessed, and rates of complication, mortality, morbidity, recurrence, and "good" clinical outcomes. **Table 2** lists the rates of surgical complications reported in various series in the literature; reported rates range from 0% to 44.8%,[12,15–25] including new onset of seizures, intraparenchymal hemorrhage, wound infection, and development of a subdural empyema. Again, a more recent meta-analysis suggests the rate of complication is likely in the range of 10.2% to 12.6%.[26] Thirty-day mortality rates are also reported in **Table 2**, with rates ranging from 0% to 20%,[12,15–19,21–25,27–30] and all cases being unrelated to intracranial pressure, focal neurologic issues, or subdural recurrence. Based on more recent and statistically elegant analyses, the actual mortality is probably closer to 4% to 6.8%.[26]

Seizures

Patients with cSDH are at risk for development of seizures, and this can have significant effects on in-hospital morbidity/mortality. Rabinstein and colleagues[31] found that in the acute (aSDH) and acute-on-chronic SDH population, rates of seizure can be as high as 25% in the immediate postoperative period. Patients in this series undergoing craniotomy were much more likely than the burr hole treatment group to experience seizures or epileptiform discharges on electroencephalogram (54.5%, P = .002), and this corresponded to a higher rate of poor outcome on discharge (P = .05), although clinical outcomes at 6 months were not significantly worse.[31] There are a few studies investigating seizure frequency and control in purely chronic SDH and even fewer that focus on craniotomy as a primary treatment modality. Grobelny and colleagues[32] found 12.5% of their cohort developed seizures related to either the subdural hematoma or the BHC, and, although preoperative AED administration did predict lower rates of seizure in a multiple logistic regression model, it did not affect outcomes at discharge. The authors manage new-onset seizures after surgery with starting an AED for a planned 6-week course and outpatient neurology follow-up for an attempt to wean the medication off. Patients with ongoing unexplained altered mental status after surgical intervention should be monitored with electroencephalogram for subclinical seizures, before or after an MRI has been obtained to rule out stroke.

POSTOPERATIVE CARE

The authors routinely monitor cSDH patients undergoing craniotomy for 1 night in the ICU for frequent neurologic examinations and a postoperative head CT. A subgaleal Jackson-Pratt drain is discontinued and mobilization on postoperative day 1 encouraged, with the assistance of physical, occupational, and speech therapies.

RECURRENCE AND CLINICAL OUTCOMES

Several retrospective studies have attempted to compare outcomes between less invasive interventions (TDC and BHC) and craniotomy. Weigel and colleagues[33] published the first evidence-based review on the topic, with a systematic review of 48 publications, demonstrating (1) higher morbidity with craniotomy compared with both TDC and BHC, (2) a nonstatistically significant trend of higher mortality with craniotomy, (3) similar cure rates between craniotomy and BHC, and (3) highest recurrence rates with TDC, suggesting that craniotomy only be used as a last resort. Subsequently, Ducruet and colleagues reviewed the topic in 2012 and performed a meta-analysis, whereby they found a statistically higher rate of complications in BHC (9.3%) compared with TDC (2.5%) and craniotomy (3.9%), although

craniotomy demonstrated a significantly higher mortality (12.2% compared with 3.7% for BHC and 5.1% for TDC). In this analysis, TDC produced statistically significantly higher recurrence rates (28.1%) compared with craniotomy (19.4%) and BHC (11.7%), although TDC also produced the highest rates of neurologic improvement (93.5% compared with 84.9% in BHC and 74.4% in craniotomy). More recently, Almenawer and colleagues[26] reviewed their experience with 834 cSDH patients and performed a meta-analysis of 34,829 patients from the literature. They concluded in a similar fashion that although craniotomy is associated with higher complication rates when used as a primary treatment strategy, it does produce better outcomes in managing recurrences compared with BHC and TDC. Craniotomy is also associated with other important costs; Regan and colleagues[25] showed that in addition to shorter hospital stay durations (which have been shown multiple times before), BHC produces shorter operating room times compared with craniotomy (78.8 vs 129.4 minutes) and less overall cost per patient ($7588 vs $10,416).

There are a tremendous number of limitations to these analyses, unfortunately, including a heterogeneous pool of patient populations with a variety of medical comorbidities and anticoagulation statuses, differences in surgical technique, cross-over, selection bias, and a lack of randomization (ie, more organized clots assigned to craniotomy). **Table 2**[12,15–25,27–30,34] summarizes the major studies in the literature to date with utilization of craniotomy with or without comparison to other forms of surgical intervention (BHC mostly) for cSDH and the reported rates of mortality and recurrence. Studies were omitted from this analysis if craniotomy as an intervention was grouped with other modalities.[35] Additionally, clinical outcome metrics are listed [in **Table 2**], with reported values for "good" outcomes [listed in **Table 2**]. All studies were retrospective in nature, with the exception that Unterhofer and colleagues[30] designed a prospective randomized trial for evaluating the role of opening the internal membranes of a cSDH.

There has been ongoing debate within literature, when a craniotomy is used, whether or not it is beneficial to surgically explore and remove the membranes associated with a cSDH (ie, a partial or complete membranectomy). Mohamed first examined this issue in 2003,[18] albeit with no other treatment group to compare outcomes to. The investigator performed an outer membranectomy only and reported no mortalities but with no information on clinical outcomes, neither immediately postoperatively nor in follow-up. Rocchi and

Table 2
Summary of previously published clinical studies of craniotomy for cSDH and definitions of "good outcomes"

Author, Year	Number of Patients with Surgery	Average Age (y)	Metric Used for Outcomes	Definition of "Good" Outcome	Surgical Modality (n)	Mortality	Recurrence with Reoperation	Other Surgical Complications (ie, Infection, Seizures, and Intracerebral Hemorrhage)	"Good" Outcome	Risk Factors for Recurrence or Worse Outcomes
Hamilton et al,[15] 1993	92	63	GOS	Good recovery	BHC (43) Crani (49)	2/43 (4.7%) 2/49 (4.1%)	3/41 (7.3%) 5/47 (10.6%)	6/41 (14.6%) 7/47 (14.9%)	66/92 (71.7%) —	None
Ernestus et al,[16] 1997	104	69 (median)	Markwalder	Neurologic improvement	BHC (94) Crani (10)	2/94 (2.1%) 2/10 (20%)	17/92 (18.5%) 1/8 (12.5%)	— —	66/92 (71.7%) 5/8 (62.5%)	Young age (<60) worse outcomes
Beatty,[17] 1999[a]	23	77	Glasgow Coma Scale	Recovery to preoperative status	Minicraniectomy (23)	2/23 (8.7%)	0	0	21/23 (91.3%) 31/33 (93.9%) 16/16 (100%)	
Tanikawa et al,[27] 2001	49	69.8 (median)	Markwalder	Stable or improved Markwalder	BHC (33) Crani (16)	1/33 (3%) 0	4/32 (12.5%) 0	— —	— —	
Mohamed[18] 2003	39	61	None	None	Crani + outer membranectomy (39)	0	0[c]	0	—	
Lee et al,[19] 2004	172	69	Markwalder	Grade 0 or 1	BHC (38) Minicrani + partial membranectomy (121) Crani + full membranectomy (13)	8/172 (4.7%)	6/38 (15.8%) 22/121 (18.2%) 3/13 (23.1%)	0 2/121 (1.7%) 0	69%	Coagulopathy was a risk factor for recurrence (41%)
Rocchi et al,[12] 2007[b]	14	62.1	None	None	Crani + full membranectomy (14)	0	0	3/14 (21.4%)	—	
Mondorf et al,[28] 2009	193	72.5	None	Symptom improvement	BHC (42) Crani (151)	1/42 (2.4%) 7/151 (4.6%)	6/42 (14.3%) 42/151 (27.8%)	— —	36/42 (85.7%) 104/151 (68.9%)	
Lindvall & Koskinen,[29] 2009	66	73.9	None	Discharge from hospital	BHC (59) Crani (7)	1/66 (1.5%) —	10/59 (16.9%) 1/7 (14.3%)	— —	65/66 (98.5%)	

Study	N	Age	Outcome Scale	Good Outcome Definition	Treatment (n)					Comments
Lee et al,[20] 2009	87	65.2 (median)	Markwalder	None	One BHC (25)	—	—	16%	—	Older age (>65 y) risk factor for recurrence; repeat operation predictive of mortality
					BHC (32)			16%		
					Minicrani (30)			3%		
White et al,[21] 2010	246	67.7	GOS	Follow-up GOS of 4 or 5, and symptom improvement (Sx)	BHC (130)	10/130 (7.7%)	23/130 (17.7%)	14/130 (10.8%)	64/77 (83.1%) GOS, 66/68 (97.1%) Sx	
					Minicraniectomy (116)	20/116 (17.2%)	23/116 (19.8%)	13/116 (11.2%)	66/90 (73.3%) GOS, 68/70 (97.1%) Sx	
Kim et al,[22] 2011	317	62.9	Markwalder	Grade 0 or 1	BHC (259)	21/259 (8.1%)	23/259 (8.9%)	9/259 (3.5%)	88%	Minicrani predictive of recurrence
					Minicrani (3 cm) + partial membranectomy (16)	0	8/16 (50%)	1/16 (6.2%)	88%	
					Crani + full membranectomy (42)	2/42 (4.8%)	4/42 (9.5%)	2/42 (4.8%)	90%	
Godlewski et al,[34] 2013[a]	42	69.7	GOS on discharge	Improved GOS	BHC (35)	—	—	13/35 (37.1%)	—	
					Crani (7)	—	—	3/7 (42.9%)	—	
Callovini et al,[23] 2014	175	71	Markwalder	Improved Markwalder	Crani + full membranectomy (34)	1/34 (2.9%)	2/34 (5.9%)	2/34 (5.9%)	89%	
Van Der Veken et al,[24] 2014	126	73	Markwalder	Improved Markwalder	Minicrani (3–4 cm)	17/126 (13.5%)	11/126 (8.7%)	8/43 (6.3%)	106/126 (84%)	Higher preoperative Markwalder predicted worse outcomes
Regan et al,[25] 2015	119	70.1	GOS, Rankin disability	Improved GOS, Rankin disability	BHC (61)	2/61 (3.3%)	4/61 (6.6%)	8/61 (13.1%)	—	
					Minicrani (5–7 cm) (58)	6/58 (6.9%)	14/58 (24.1%)	26/58 (44.8%)	—	
Unterhofer et al,[30] 2016	57	72	Markwalder	None	Minicrani (3 cm) (28)	0	6/28 (21.4%)	—	—	
					Minicrani + inner membranectomy (28)	0	8/28 (28.6%)	—	—	

[a] Only cSDH analyzed (not aSDH or subacute SDH).
[b] Only 5 patients treated with upfront craniotomy; remainder were recurrence after BHC or TDC.
[c] 2/39 or 5.1% required percutaneous bedside tap.

colleagues[12] performed a similar, limited report of craniotomy with full membranectomy in a limited number of patients, with no mortalities or recurrence; however, they did have a relatively high complication rate (21.4%). Callovini and colleagues[23] provide the most thorough validation of the craniotomy with a full membranectomy, reporting a complication and recurrence rate of 5.9%. Again, the results are limited, because there are no comparison groups, and there is an inherent selection bias for cSDH with evidence of septations and membranes. Lee and colleagues[19] compared full and partial membranectomy to BHC. This study demonstrated for the first time that the highest recurrence rates were with full-membranectomy, with preoperative coagulopathy demonstrating a strong association with recurrence. Complication rates were similar among the 3 groups, and mortality and clinical outcomes were reasonable, although not analyzed in relation to the surgical approach. Kim and colleagues,[22] in contrast, found higher rates of recurrence with the minicraniotomy and partial membranectomy, with similar rates of morbidity and efficacy among the 3 operative approaches. Finally, Unterhofer and colleagues[30] recently and convincingly demonstrated no benefit of membranectomy to decreasing recurrence rates, because this was done in a randomized, prospective fashion.

There are a variety of clinical outcomes that are reported in cSDH series, although the Markwalder scale (see **Table 1**) and Glasgow Outcome Scale (GOS) seem the most commonly used. Both improvements in Markwalder grade and a Markwalder grade of 0 or 1 are typically considered "good outcomes," although there is a definite need for a more unified opinion on the topic, to help enable comparisons across studies. Positive outcomes are reported in craniotomy in a range from 62.5% to 100%, compared with 71.1% to 97.1% with BHC. There seems to be equipoise in terms of efficacy between the 2 modalities.[30]

SUMMARY

Craniotomy remains a viable, safe, and effective tool for treating cSDH in cases of recurrence or as an upfront modality with radiographic evidence of intrahematoma septations and membranes. Direct comparison to BHC and other surgical modalities is difficult, because all prior reports in the literature harbor fundamental selection bias, although efficacy seems comparable, with a slightly higher rate of mortality, morbidity, and recurrence, when compared at a glance. Full membranectomy does not reduce recurrence rates. Minicraniectomy is another viable subtype of craniotomy, although there are obvious concerns with postoperative cosmesis and a sunken appearance on the scalp. Future studies should aim for (1) prospective and randomized design and (2) consistency with defining and measuring clinical outcomes.

REFERENCES

1. Fogelholm R, Heiskanen O, Waltimo O. Chronic subdural hematoma in adults. Influence of patient's age on symptoms, signs, and thickness of hematoma. J Neurosurg 1975;42(1):43–6.
2. Huang KT, Bi WL, Abd-El-Barr M, et al. The neurocritical and neurosurgical care of subdural hematomas. Neurocrit Care 2016;24(2):294–307.
3. Tokmak M, Iplikcioglu AC, Bek S, et al. The role of exudation in chronic subdural hematomas. J Neurosurg 2007;107(2):290–5.
4. Lee KS. Natural history of chronic subdural haematoma. Brain Inj 2004;18(4):351–8.
5. Markwalder TM, Steinsiepe KF, Rohner M, et al. The course of chronic subdural hematomas after burrhole craniostomy and closed-system drainage. J Neurosurg 1981;55(3):390–6.
6. Nomura S, Kashiwagi S, Fujisawa H, et al. Characterization of local hyperfibrinolysis in chronic subdural hematomas by SDS-PAGE and immunoblot. J Neurosurg 1994;81(6):910–3.
7. Delgado-Lopez PD, Martin-Velasco V, Castilla-Diez JM, et al. Dexamethasone treatment in chronic subdural haematoma. Neurocirugia (Astur) 2009; 20(4):346–59.
8. Ducruet AF, Grobelny BT, Zacharia BE, et al. The surgical management of chronic subdural hematoma. Neurosurg Rev 2012;35(2):155–69 [discussion: 169].
9. Ivamoto HS, Lemos HP, Atallah AN. Surgical treatments for chronic subdural hematomas: a comprehensive systematic review. World Neurosurg 2016; 86:399–410.
10. Gjerris F, Schmidt K. Chronic subdural hematoma. Surgery or mannitol treatment. J Neurosurg 1974; 40(5):639–42.
11. Lega BC, Danish SF, Malhotra NR, et al. Choosing the best operation for chronic subdural hematoma: a decision analysis. J Neurosurg 2010;113(3):615–21.
12. Rocchi G, Caroli E, Salvati M, et al. Membranectomy in organized chronic subdural hematomas: indications and technical notes. Surg Neurol 2007;67(4): 374–80 [discussion: 380].
13. Asfora WT, Schwebach L. A modified technique to treat chronic and subacute subdural hematoma: technical note. Surg Neurol 2003;59(4):329–32 [discussion: 332].
14. Chari A, Kolias AG, Santarius T, et al. Twist-drill craniostomy with hollow screws for evacuation of

chronic subdural hematoma. J Neurosurg 2014;
121(1):176–83.

15. Hamilton MG, Frizzell JB, Tranmer BI. Chronic subdural hematoma: the role for craniotomy reevaluated. Neurosurgery 1993;33(1):67–72.

16. Ernestus RI, Beldzinski P, Lanfermann H, et al. Chronic subdural hematoma: surgical treatment and outcome in 104 patients. Surg Neurol 1997; 48(3):220–5.

17. Beatty RA. Subdural haematomas in the elderly: experience with treatment by trephine craniotomy and not closing the dura or replacing the bone plate. Br J Neurosurg 1999;13(1):60–4.

18. Mohamed EE. Chronic subdural haematoma treated by craniotomy, durectomy, outer membranectomy and subgaleal suction drainage. Personal experience in 39 patients. Br J Neurosurg 2003;17(3): 244–7.

19. Lee JY, Ebel H, Ernestus RI, et al. Various surgical treatments of chronic subdural hematoma and outcome in 172 patients: is membranectomy necessary? Surg Neurol 2004;61(6):523–7 [discussion: 527–8].

20. Lee JK, Choi JK, Kim CH, et al. Chronic subdural hematomas: a comparative study of three types of operative procedures. J Korean Neurosurg Soc 2009;46(3):210–4.

21. White M, Mathieson CS, Campbell E, et al. Treatment of chronic subdural haematomas - a retrospective comparison of minicraniectomy versus burrhole drainage. Br J Neurosurg 2010;24(3):257–60.

22. Kim JH, Kang DS, Kim JH, et al. Chronic subdural hematoma treated by small or large craniotomy with membranectomy as the initial treatment. J Korean Neurosurg Soc 2011;50(2):103–8.

23. Callovini GM, Bolognini A, Callovini G, et al. Primary enlarged craniotomy in organized chronic subdural hematomas. Neurol Med Chir (Tokyo) 2014;54(5): 349–56.

24. Van Der Veken J, Duerinck J, Buyl R, et al. Minicraniotomy as the primary surgical intervention for the treatment of chronic subdural hematoma–a retrospective analysis. Acta Neurochir (Wien) 2014; 156(5):981–7.

25. Regan JM, Worley E, Shelburne C, et al. Burr hole washout versus craniotomy for chronic subdural

hematoma: patient outcome and cost analysis. PLoS One 2015;10(1):e0115085.

26. Almenawer SA, Farrokhyar F, Hong C, et al. Chronic subdural hematoma management: a systematic review and meta-analysis of 34,829 patients. Ann Surg 2014;259(3):449–57.

27. Tanikawa M, Mase M, Yamada K, et al. Surgical treatment of chronic subdural hematoma based on intrahematomal membrane structure on MRI. Acta Neurochir (Wien) 2001;143(6):613–8 [discussion: 618–9].

28. Mondorf Y, Abu-Owaimer M, Gaab MR, et al. Chronic subdural hematoma–craniotomy versus burr hole trepanation. Br J Neurosurg 2009;23(6):612–6.

29. Lindvall P, Koskinen L. Anticoagulants and antiplatelet agents and the risk of development and recurrence of chronic subdural haematomas. J Clin Neurosci 2009;16(10):1287–90.

30. Unterhofer C, Freyschlag CF, Thome C, et al. Opening the internal hematoma membrane does not alter the recurrence rate of chronic subdural hematomas - a prospective randomized trial. World Neurosurg 2016;92:31–6.

31. Rabinstein AA, Chung SY, Rudzinski LA, et al. Seizures after evacuation of subdural hematomas: incidence, risk factors, and functional impact. J Neurosurg 2010;112(2):455–60.

32. Grobelny BT, Ducruet AF, Zacharia BE, et al. Preoperative antiepileptic drug administration and the incidence of postoperative seizures following bur hole-treated chronic subdural hematoma. J Neurosurg 2009; 111(6):1257–62.

33. Weigel R, Schmiedek P, Krauss JK. Outcome of contemporary surgery for chronic subdural haematoma: evidence based review. J Neurol Neurosurg Psychiatry 2003;74(7):937–43.

34. Godlewski B, Pawelczyk A, Pawelczyk T, et al. Retrospective analysis of operative treatment of a series of 100 patients with subdural hematoma. Neurol Med Chir (Tokyo) 2013;53(1):26–33.

35. Horn EM, Feiz-Erfan I, Bristol RE, et al. Bedside twist drill craniostomy for chronic subdural hematoma: a comparative study. Surg Neurol 2006;65(2):150–3 [discussion: 153–4].

Chronic Subdural Hematoma ICU Management

Jeremy T. Ragland, MD, Kiwon Lee, MD*

KEYWORDS

- Chronic subdural hematoma • ICU • Cerebral spinal fluid • Anticoagulants • Antiplatelet agents

KEY POINTS

- A chronic subdural hematoma (cSDH) is a collection of old (>3 weeks) blood products and blood breakdown products that have accumulated in the subdural space, which is a potential space between the dura mater and the arachnoid layers of the meninges.
- cSDH is increasingly common due to the combination of more frequent use of anticoagulant and antiplatelet agents and the advanced age of many people in the population.
- The incidence of cSDH is estimated to be between 3.4 and 58 per 100,000 person-years, depending on the age of the population, with the average presenting age 63 years.
- The United Nations predicts that the percentage of the population above the age of 65 is expected to double between 2010 and 2050.
- cSDH is more prevalent in men, with a 3:1 male-to-female ratio.

CASE PRESENTATION

A 50-year-old man with a history of hypertension and alcohol abuse with prior withdrawal-related seizures presented to an outside hospital facility with confusion and headache after a witnessed fall. Further questioning revealed that he suffered a fall approximately 8 weeks prior to presentation. Since then he has been experiencing progressive dizziness and intermittent headaches. For the 10 days prior to presentation, he noticed progressive right arm weakness. On the day of presentation, after drinking a few beers, bystanders noted that he was confused and then suffered a fall from standing without head strike or loss of consciousness. The emergency medical service was activated, and he was taken to an outside hospital facility for evaluation. Initial vital signs were notable for no fever with blood pressure 152/105 mm Hg and a pulse of 102 beats per minute. He was awake and alert but confused. He was able to state his name and provide the history surrounding his fall but was unable to state his current location or the date. He was very combative. His right pupil was 6 mm and left pupil was 5 mm and both were reactive to light. He had pronator and downward drift in the right arm with decreased strength in all muscle groups. He had full strength in the left arm and both legs. His Glasgow Coma Scale (GCS) score was 14. His initial blood testing was notable for normal electrolytes, slightly elevated liver function tests, and mild anemia with normal platelet count and normal coagulation studies. CT scan of the head showed large left-sided cSDH (**Fig. 1**). He was immediately transported to the authors' facility for further management.

Departments of Neurosurgery and Neurology, Division of Neurocritical Care McGovern Medical School, 6431 Fannin Street, Medical School Building 7.152, University of Texas Health Science Center at Houston, Houston, TX 77030, USA
* Corresponding author.
E-mail address: kiwon.lee@uth.tmc.edu

Neurosurg Clin N Am 28 (2017) 239–246
http://dx.doi.org/10.1016/j.nec.2016.11.006

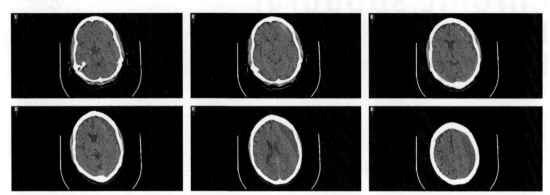

Fig. 1. Patient's initial CT scan. Non–contrast-enhanced CT scan of the head showing an acute-on-chronic left subdural hematoma with a maximum thickness of 2.4 cm and 7 mm of left-to-right midline shift.

INTRODUCTION

A cSDH is a collection of old (>3 weeks) blood products and blood breakdown products that have accumulated in the subdural space, which is a potential space between the dura mater and the arachnoid layers of the meninges.[1] cSDH is increasingly common due to the combination of more frequent use of anticoagulant and antiplatelet agents and the advanced age of many people in the population.[2] The incidence of cSDH is estimated to be between 3.4 and 58 per 100,000 person-years, depending on the age of the population.[1,3–6] The average presenting age is 63 years.[6] The United Nations predicts that the percentage of the population above the age of 65 is expected to double between 2010 and 2050.[2] The US census reported that 12% of the population (or 35.9 million people) were over the age of 65 in 2003. This is expected to rise to approximately 20% of the population (or 72 million people) by the year 2030.[7] The incidence of cSDH is expected to follow accordingly. In elderly individuals, cSDH has been identified as a sentinel event linked to underlying systemic pathology with 1-year mortality similar to that of a hip fracture.[2] cSDH is more prevalent in men, with a 3:1 male-to-female ratio.[2,3,8,9] cSDH is bilateral in 20% to 25% of cases.[6]

cSDH occurs at the dural border cell layer, which is between the dura mater and arachnoid mater (**Fig. 2**).[1,2,7] Generally, 2 predisposing factors must be present for a cSDH to develop: (1) decreased brain volume (eg, in elderly patients and patients abusing alcohol) and (2) previous head trauma.[2,7] Experts believe there are several causes that lead to the formation of cSDH. The 2 most common are thought to be an acute subdural hematoma and a subdural hygroma (a collection of cerebral spinal fluid in the subdural space).[1,2,6,7] In

acute subdural hematoma, incomplete resorption of the blood products leads to the formation of cSDH. In both causes, a substantial inflammatory response infiltrates the subdural space. This inflammation includes angiogenic factors that lead to neovascularization. Although these friable capillaries are forming, they are subject to microhemorrhages, which result in cSDH. Many risk factors are thought to contribute to the formation of cSDH, including advanced age, history of falls, alcohol abuse (due to brain atrophy, increased fall risk, and coagulopathy), epilepsy, low intracranial pressure states, and hemodialysis.[1,2] As discussed previously, there has been an increase in the use of anticoagulants and antiplatelet agents. This has led to a higher incidence of both atraumatic cSDH (whereby the antecedent trauma is so minor that it is not recalled) and recurrent cSDH.[2]

Some sources refer to cSDH as the "great imitator" given its heterogenous presenting symptoms and that its symptom onset can range from days to weeks prior to presentation.[2,10] In a pooled cohort of 205 randomized controlled trial participants, presenting symptoms included gait disturbance and falls, cognitive decline, limb weakness, and acute confusion (**Box 1**).[8] In the same cohort, a majority of patients presented with a GCS score 13 to 15 (81%) whereas 12% had a GCS score 9 to 12, and 7% had a GCS score less than or equal to 8.[8] A diagnosis of cSDH is usually made using CT scan of the head, on which cSDH usually appears as a hypodense, crescent-shaped collection along the convexity of the brain.[1,2,7] There may be the presence of hyperdense or isodense material associated with the hypodense collection owing to the descriptive terms, acute-on-chronic hematoma and subacute-on-chronic subdural hematoma, respectively.[11]

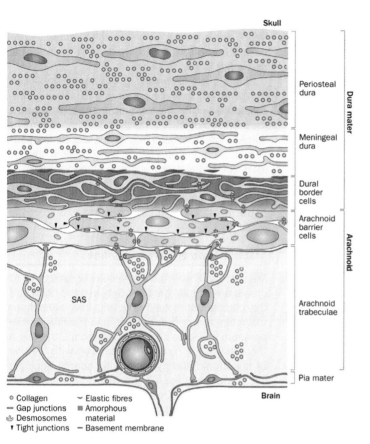

Skull

Periosteal dura

Meningeal dura

Dural border cells

Arachnoid barrier cells

Arachnoid trabeculae

Pia mater

Brain

Dura mater

Arachnoid

SAS

○ Collagen   ～ Elastic fibres
— Gap junctions   ■ Amorphous
⚓ Desmosomes   material
▼ Tight junctions   — Basement membrane

Fig. 2. Schematic of the ultrastructure of the meninges. SAS, subarachnoid space. (*Adapted from* Haines DED. On the question of a subdural space. Anat Rec 1991;230(1):3–21; with permission.)

PREOPERATIVE MANAGEMENT

Initial assessment of a patient with a cSDH should include evaluations of the airway, breathing, and circulation. Any acutely life-threatening issues should be appropriately managed. As a general rule, a GCS score of less than 8 warrants endotracheal intubation. A detailed history should be obtained with a focus on prior falls and head trauma as well as the use of antiplatelet or anticoagulant agents. A physical examination should be conducted, including a calculation of GCS score and evaluation for focal neurologic deficits. Initial laboratory evaluation should include chemistries and electrolytes, complete blood cell count, liver function tests, and coagulation studies. A noncontrast CT scan of the head should be completed to make a diagnosis of cSDH.[1,2,7]

Reversal of Coagulopathies

Once the patient is stabilized, the focus should move to the management of any coagulopathies. The initial step is the cessation of any anticoagulant or antiplatelet agents. The next step is the decision to reverse any coagulopathy that may

exist. One series of 88 patients showed that patients with cSDH who presented on anticoagulant medications experienced a significantly longer hospital stay (11 vs 7.5 days, $P = .040$), although the percentage with a good modified Rankin scale at discharge was not significantly different between the groups.[7] General consensus is that patients with cSDH presenting on anticoagulant medications should undergo rapid reversal to prevent hematoma expansion and to allow for urgent neurosurgical intervention; this even applies to patients on anticoagulation for prosthetic heart valves.[7,12] Oral warfarin, a vitamin K antagonist, is the most frequently used anticoagulant medication associated with cSDH.[13] The vitamin K antagonists are reversed using prothrombin complex concentrate (PCC), fresh frozen plasma (FFP), and vitamin K.[14,15] Traditionally, FFP has been the first-line therapy in the reversal of vitamin K antagonists. Its use, however, can predispose to additional medical complications given its large volume of infusion.[7,15,16] Alternatively, PCC can be infused over a few minutes and has a volume exponentially smaller than FFP.[7,15,17] With both PCC and FFP, vitamin K should be used an adjunctive therapy to facilitate the liver in producing new clotting factors.[15] For cases in which a more gradual reversal technique is acceptable, vitamin K can be used as monotherapy.[12] Most institutions have guidelines on the use of these agents. The clinical situation and the acuity of any necessary surgical intervention guide the decision on which agents to use.

Novel oral anticoagulants (NOACs) include factor Xa inhibitors and direct thrombin inhibitors. There is limited experience with the reversal of these agents. The best antidote for NOACs is time in the absence of life-threatening acute hematoma expansion or the need for emergent surgical intervention. The Neurocritical Care Society guidelines suggest using activated charcoal and PCC for NOAC reversal, but this is based on low-quality evidence and this decision should be made with input from a hematologist.[15] The direct thrombin inhibitor dabigatran now has a Food and Drug Administration–approved antidote, idarucizumab. It is suggested that the reversal of dabigatran involve activated charcoal, hemodialysis, and PCC (all low-quality evidence) and idarucizumab (moderate-quality evidence).[15] Laboratory assays have been developed that can aid in assessing the anticoagulant effect of NOACs. Diluted

thrombin time for direct thrombin inhibitors and factor Xa levels for factor Xa inhibitors are inconsistently available and the extent of their clinical use is not fully established.[18]

For antiplatelet therapy, it has been established that 7 to 10 days are necessary to allow for the production of fully functional platelets to replace the inhibited ones in circulation.[19] When emergent surgical intervention is necessary, platelet transfusion is recommended to acutely reverse the effects of antiplatelet agents although there is scant evidence to support this.[20] Some centers combine platelet transfusion with a single dose of desmopressin, but this too is based on minimal evidence.[21]

Mannitol and Hypertonic Saline

Mannitol and hypertonic saline are agents used to create an osmotic gradient between the brain and the plasma, ultimately removing free water from the brain in an effort to decrease the intracranial pressure. In acute subdural hematoma, there is a theoretic concern of SDH expansion with the use of hypertonic and hyperosmotic agents because it is thought that the full brain has a tamponade effect on the SDH. Despite this theoretic concern, the temporary use of hypertonic and hyperosmotic agents in patients actively experiencing cerebral herniation or impending herniation should be advocated as a temporizing measure prior to surgical intervention.

Seizure Prophylaxis

Only a few studies have examined the rate of seizures in patients with cSDH.[22–25] The preoperative incidence of seizures ranged from 2% to 19%; postoperative seizure incidence was 1% to 23%.[2,7] Two studies reported no significant difference in the seizure rate related to the use of prophylactic anticonvulsive medications (ACMs).[7,23,24] The investigators concluded that there was no benefit in using prophylactic ACM except in patients at high risk of seizures, such as patients abusing alcohol.[23,24] A third study showed that 2.4% of patients treated with therapeutic prophylactic ACMs experienced a seizures compared with 32% of patients who were not adequately treated with prophylactic ACMs.[25] The investigators concluded that this significantly increased the morbidity and mortality for the patients who experienced new-onset seizures and therefore recommended the use of prophylactic ACMs in cSDH.[25] A fourth study found that preoperative administration of prophylactic ACMs was the only independent predictor of decreased incidence of postoperative seizures.[22] Despite this, there was no effect on discharge outcomes, suggesting that, if given, prophylactic ACMs should be administered prior to surgical intervention.[7] Given these mixed results, practices vary in their use of prophylactic ACMs. The authors' practice is to treat with seizure prophylaxis for 7 days, especially in patients who are undergoing surgical intervention or have an increased risk of seizures, such as alcoholics or those with significant underlying traumatic brain injury.

Corticosteroids

Because inflammation plays a role in the pathophysiology of cSDH, multiple studies have examined the use of corticosteroids as monotherapy to avoid surgery and in combination to surgical intervention.[26–30] Medical management of cSDH is discussed in a See Jan Claassen's article, "Chronic Subdural Medical Management", in this issue, so monotherapy is not discussed in this article. European studies have shown the use of preoperative and postoperative steroids reduces the rate of cSDH recurrence after surgical treatment and decreases 6-month mortality.[2,28] An additional retrospective study suggests that local application of methylprednisolone into the hematoma cavity at the time of surgery may reduce hematoma recurrence.[31] The evidence is insufficient, however, to draw any significant conclusions, and further study with randomized controlled trials should be conducted. It is the authors' practice not to use steroids as monotherapy or as adjunctive therapy to surgical intervention in the treatment of cSDH. The use of corticosteroids in the treatment of cSDH is generally not recommended due to lack of evidence.

Indication for Surgical Intervention

Clinical presentation and radiographic appearance both influence the decision for surgical intervention. A small cSDH in an asymptomatic patient is best managed with clinical and radiographic observation in a closely monitored setting.[1,7] Should a patient develop significant neurologic symptoms, however, surgical intervention is advised.[1,2] Although the radiographic size of the cSDH plays a role in the decision for surgery, there is no absolute size greater than which a surgical intervention is mandated.[1,7] The spontaneous resolution of cSDHs of significant size has been reported in a few case series.[1,7,32,33] The investigators described these patients as advanced in age (>70 years) with significant cerebral atrophy and no clinical or radiographic evidence of increased intracranial pressure.[32,33]

Management of asymptomatic patients with cSDHs large enough to cause brain compression and/or midline shift remains a controversial topic. Despite the lack of evidence to establish a size cutoff, it is generally accepted that hematoma volume with a maximum thickness greater than 1 cm, or greater than the thickness of the skull, should undergo surgical evacuation.[1,6]

Patients with neurologic symptoms that can be attributed to a radiographically proved cSDH warrant immediate surgical evacuation. These symptoms are dictated by the location of the cSDH but can include aphasia, neglect, contralateral hemiparesis, and partial seizures. For patients with a large cSDH causing mass effect on the left frontotemporal convexity, it is not uncommon to observe a profound aphasia; some of these patients have severe global aphasia with or without contralateral hemiparesis. An isolated aphasia with intact level of alertness is often due to the chemical irritation of the dominant hemisphere and does not necessarily mean the patient is experiencing a stroke or status epilepticus. Although it is prudent to rule out acute ischemic stroke and seizures for anyone with acute aphasia, such a symptom is frequently seen with dominant hemispheric convexity subdural hematomas — whether acute or chronic. Large hematomas, or those in a frontotemporal location, can lead to brainstem compression resulting in anisocoria, coma, and death. The presence of these symptoms associated with a cSDH necessitates emergent surgical intervention. Surgical options include burr hole craniostomy, twist drill craniostomy, and craniotomy, all of which are discussed in See William Mack's article, "Minimally Invasive Surgical Approaches for Chronic Subdural Hematomas and See Louis Kim's article, Craniotomy for treatment of chronic subdural hematoma", in this issue.

POSTOPERATIVE MANAGEMENT
Postoperative Imaging

The timing and frequency of postoperative CT scans in cSDH are topics of controversy. Practitioners must weigh the advantage of daily CT scans (objective monitoring of the cSDH drainage) versus the disadvantages (radiation exposure to patients and health care costs). One study used early (within 48 hours) postoperative CT to predict outcome at discharge.[34] Because it found that (1) the only predictive factor of postoperative SDH volume was preoperative SDH volume and (2) early postoperative SDH volume on CT did not correlate with outcome at discharge, the investigators concluded that routine postoperative CT scan may be unnecessary.[34] In the authors' practice, a CT scan of the head is completed 24 hours after operative intervention. A second routine CT scan is performed just prior to planned removal of the subdural drain unless the patient has a clinical change or there is an issue with the drainage catheter output. Obtaining daily scans for a patient who is neurologically doing well is of low yield and generally not recommended.

Mobilization

The timing of mobilization after surgical treatment of cSDH remains a controversial issue. Although early mobilization decreases the risk of medical complications, its benefit has to be weighed against the risk of recurrent cSDH, which is thought to be prevented by bed rest.[7] Practices vary with regards to early mobilization versus prolonged bed rest. One study using historical controls showed significantly fewer medical complications with early mobilization (postoperative day 1) compared with delayed mobilization (postoperative day 3) although there was no difference in the rate of recurrence.[35] A second study also found no significant difference in the rate of recurrence between patients who remained recumbent for 3 days postoperatively compared with those who assumed a sitting position on postoperative day 1.[36] Alternatively, a third study examined elevating the head of bed to 30° to 40° compared with strict supine position in the first 3 postoperative days and showed a significant reduction in the rate of recurrent cSDH in the strict supine group (19% vs 2.3%).[37] There was no significant difference in other position-related medical complications, including pneumonia, atelectasis, deep vein thrombosis, and decubitus ulcers.[37]

Venous Thromboembolism Prophylaxis

Patients with cSDH are at risk for complications related to venous thromboembolism (VTE). Unless contraindicated, all patients should have intermittent pneumatic compression devices placed on their legs. There is controversy surrounding the use of chemical VTE prophylaxis. One study showed an increase in recurrence of cSDH after the use of a prophylactic dose of low-molecular-weight heparin (18.8% vs 32.1%) although it is unclear from the study on what postoperative day the prophylaxis was started.[38] A separate institution recommends starting chemical VTE prophylaxis only after the closed drainage system has been removed and there is a follow-up CT scan showing no acute or recurrent hemorrhage.[7] Despite this, many ICUs routinely start chemical

VTE prophylaxis 24 to 72 hours after surgical intervention.[2] More studies are needed to examine the ideal time to start chemical VTE prophylaxis after surgery and to compare the risks and benefits of low-molecular-weight heparin with unfractionated heparin. It is reasonable to use chemical VTE prophylaxis starting 24 hours after operative intervention for cSDH in stable patients.

Resuming Antiplatelet and Anticoagulant Agents

Many patients with cSDH are also taking antiplatelet and anticoagulant agents. Because these agents are generally taken to prevent heart disease and ischemic stroke, there is pressure on practitioners to restart these medications as early as safely possible. There are varying opinions on not only when to restart these medications but also whether the doses should be adjusted on restarting. Currently these decisions are made on a patient-by-patient basis.[2] Variables that should be considered are patient age, indication for antiplatelet or anticoagulant agents, risk for future falls and head trauma, and underlying cause of cSDH. Comparison between CHA2DS2-VASc score and HAS-BLED score can provide some objective data to aid in the decision of restarting warfarin in patients with atrial fibrillation.[39–41] The CHA2DS2-VASc score evaluates the risk for cerebral thromboembolic events in patients with atrial fibrillation, and the HAS-BLED score estimates the risk of major bleeding in patients on anticoagulation for atrial fibrillation.[40,41] Limited data suggest safety in restarting warfarin 72 hours after surgical intervention. There are sparse data when it comes to the use of NOACs.

Case Summary

The authors' patient was admitted to the neuroscience ICU. Valproic acid was started for seizure prophylaxis. The cSDH was managed with burr hole craniostomy and closed drainage system completed in the operating room. His postoperative course was complicated by alcohol withdrawal requiring high doses of benzodiazepines. After adequate drainage, the subdural drain was removed. He was discharged to a rehabilitation facility after recovering from alcohol withdrawal.

REFERENCES

1. Soleman J, Taussky P, Fandino J, et al. Evidence-based treatment of chronic subdural hematoma. In: Sadaka F, editor. Traumatic brain injury. Rijeka(Croatia); 2014. p. 249–81.

2. Kolias AG. Chronic subdural haematoma: modern management and emerging therapies. Nat Rev Neurol 2014;10(10):570–8.

3. Cousseau DH. Chronic and subacute subdural haematoma. An epidemiological study in a captive population. Rev Neurol 2001;32(9):821–4 [in Spanish].

4. Asghar MM. Chronic subdural haematoma in the elderly–a North Wales experience. J R Soc Med 2002;95(6):290–2.

5. Kudo HH. Chronic subdural hematoma in elderly people: present status on Awaji Island and epidemiological prospect. Neurol Med Chir (Tokyo) 1992;32(4):207–9.

6. Greenberg M. Chronic subdural hematoma. Handbook of neurosurgery. 3rd edition. New York: Thieme; 2010. p. 899–902.

7. Ducruet AF. The surgical management of chronic subdural hematoma. Neurosurg Rev 2012;35(2):155–69.

8. Santarius T, Kirkpatrick PJ, Ganesan D, et al. Use of drains versus no drains after burr-hole evacuation of chronic subdural haematoma: a randomised controlled trial. Lancet 2009;374(9695):1067–73.

9. Gelabert-González M. Chronic subdural haematoma: surgical treatment and outcome in 1000 cases. Clin Neurol Neurosurg 2005;107(3):223–9.

10. Potter JF. Chronic subdural hematoma–the "great imitator". Geriatrics 1977;32(6):61–6.

11. Yousem DM. Head trauma. Neuroradiology: the requisites. 3rd edition. Philadelphia: Elsevier Health Sciences; 2010. p. 173–6.

12. Hanley JP. Warfarin reversal. J Clin Pathol 2004;57(11):1132–9.

13. Ansell J. The pharmacology and management of the vitamin K antagonists. Chest 2004;126(3):204S–33S.

14. Cartmill MM. Prothrombin complex concentrate for oral anticoagulant reversal in neurosurgical emergencies. Br J Neurosurg 2000;14(5):458–61.

15. Frontera JA. Guideline for reversal of antithrombotics in intracranial hemorrhage a statement for healthcare professionals from the neurocritical care society and society of critical care medicine. Neurocrit Care 2015;24(1):6–46.

16. Lankiewicz MW. Urgent reversal of warfarin with prothrombin complex concentrate. J Thromb Haemost 2006;4(5):967–70.

17. Vigué B. Ultra-rapid management of oral anticoagulant therapy-related surgical intracranial hemorrhage. Intensive Care Med 2007;33(4):721–5.

18. Heidbuchel H. Updated European Heart Rhythm Association practical guide on the use of non-vitamin-K antagonist anticoagulants in patients with non-valvular atrial fibrillation: executive summary. Eur Heart J 2016;17:1467–507.

19. Wada M. Influence of antiplatelet therapy on postoperative recurrence of chronic subdural hematoma: a multicenter retrospective study in 719 patients. Clin Neurol Neurosurg 2014;120:49–54.

20. Handin RI. Hemostatic effectiveness of platelets stored at 22°C. N Engl J Med 1971;285(10):538–43.

21. Ranucci M. Platelet mapping and desmopressin reversal of platelet inhibition during emergency carotid endarterectomy. J Cardiothorac Vasc Anesth 2007;21(6):851–4.

22. Grobelny BT. Preoperative antiepileptic drug administration and the incidence of postoperative seizures following bur hole–treated chronic subdural hematoma Clinical article. J Neurosurg 2009;111(6):1257–62.

23. Ohno KK. Low incidence of seizures in patients with chronic subdural haematoma. J Neurol Neurosurg And Psychiatry 1993;56(11):1231–3.

24. Rubin GG. Epilepsy in chronic subdural haematoma. Acta Neurochir (Wien) 1993;123(1–2):39–42.

25. Sabo RA. Chronic subdural hematomas and seizures: the role of prophylactic anticonvulsive medication. Surg Neurol 1995;43(6):579–82.

26. Frati A. Inflammation markers and risk factors for recurrence in 35 patients with a posttraumatic chronic subdural hematoma: a prospective study. J Neurosurg 2004;100(1):24–32.

27. Santarius TT. Working toward rational and evidence-based treatment of chronic subdural hematoma. Clin Neurosurg 2010;57:112–22.

28. Berghauser Pont LM, Dammers R, Schouten JW, et al. Clinical factors associated with outcome in chronic subdural hematoma: a retrospective cohort study of patients on preoperative corticosteroid therapy. Neurosurgery 2012;70(4):873–80.

29. Sun TF, Boet R, Poon WS. Non-surgical primary treatment of chronic subdural haematoma: preliminary results of using dexamethasone. Br J Neurosurg 2005;19(4):327–33.

30. Berghauser Pont LM, Dirven CM, Dippel DW. The role of corticosteroids in the management of chronic subdural hematoma: a systematic review. Eur J Neurol 2012;19(11):1397–403.

31. Xu X. Local application of corticosteroids combined with surgery for the treatment of chronic subdural hematoma. Turk Neurosurg 2013;25(2):252–5.

32. Göksu EE. Spontaneous resolution of a large chronic subdural hematoma: a case report and review of the literature. Ulusal Travma Acil Cerrahi Derg 2009;15(1):95–8.

33. Parlato CC. Spontaneous resolution of chronic subdural hematoma. Surg Neurol 2000;53(4):312–5 [discussion: 315–7].

34. Ng HY. Value of routine early post-operative computed tomography in determining short-term functional outcome after drainage of chronic subdural hematoma: an evaluation of residual volume. Surg Neurol Int 2014;5(1):136.

35. Kurabe S. Efficacy and safety of postoperative early mobilization for chronic subdural hematoma in elderly patients. Acta Neurochir (Wien) 2010;152(7):1171–4.

36. Nakajima HH. The role of postoperative patient posture in the recurrence of chronic subdural hematoma: a prospective randomized trial. Surg Neurol 2002;58(6):385–7 [discussion: 387].

37. Abouzari M. The role of postoperative patient posture in the recurrence of traumatic chronic subdural hematoma after burr-hole surgery. Neurosurgery 2007;61(4):794–7.

38. Tahsim-Oglou Y. Factors predicting recurrence of chronic subdural haematoma: the influence of intraoperative irrigation and low-molecular-weight heparin thromboprophylaxis. Acta Neurochir (Wien) 2012;154(6):1063–8.

39. Chari A. Recommencement of anticoagulation in chronic subdural haematoma: a systematic review and meta-analysis. Br J Neurosurg 2014; 28(1):2–7.

40. Olesen JB. Risks of thromboembolism and bleeding with thromboprophylaxis in patients with atrial fibrillation: a net clinical benefit analysis using a 'real world' nationwide cohort study. Thromb Haemost 2011;106(4):739–49.

41. Pisters RA. Novel user-friendly score (HAS-BLED) to assess 1-year risk of major bleeding in patients with atrial fibrillation. Chest 2010;138(5):1093–100.

Natural History of Acute Subdural Hematoma

Rafael A. Vega, MD, PhD, Alex B. Valadka, MD*

KEYWORDS

- Acute subdural hematoma • Anticoagulation • Computed tomography • Glasgow coma scale • MRI
- Nonoperative management • Traumatic brain injury

KEY POINTS

- Although guidelines for surgical decision-making in patients with acute subdural hematomas (ASDHs) are widely available, the evidence supporting these guidelines is weak, and management of these patients must often be individualized.
- Smaller ASDHs in patients in good neurologic condition usually can be successfully managed without surgery.
- Large ASDHs with minimal mass effect in patients with minimal symptoms also may be considered for nonoperative management.
- The literature is divided about the effects of anticoagulant and antiplatelet medications on rapid growth of ASDHs and on their likelihood of progression to large chronic subdural hematomas, but it is reasonable to reverse the effects of these medications promptly.
- Close clinical and radiologic follow-up is needed in these patients, both acutely to detect rapid expansion of an ASDH, and subacutely to detect formation of a large subacute or chronic subdural hematoma.

INTRODUCTION

Few emergencies in neurosurgery are as worrisome as a large acute subdural hematoma (ASDH) (**Fig. 1**). Many of these lesions require immediate evacuation, regardless of the time of day or day of the week. Fortunately for the affected patients, the vast majority of ASDHs are relatively small, thus allowing initial management to consist of nonsurgical observation.

The decision that emergency surgery is not needed is soon followed by an obvious question: what will happen to the ASDH? The ideal scenario is that it will gradually resorb and the patient will be left with no deficits. But the worst-case scenario is rapid and unexpected enlargement of the hematoma, causing the patient to undergo neurologic deterioration and immediate surgical evacuation. Over a more protracted course, another suboptimal outcome is progression of a small ASDH to a large chronic subdural hematoma (CSDH) (**Figs. 2 and 3**), which may enlarge to such an extent that surgical evacuation becomes necessary (**Fig. 4**).

Despite the frequency with which neurosurgeons have to make these decisions, and despite the likely increase in incidence of small but potentially worrisome ASDHs as the population ages, becomes more prone to falls, and consumes more antiplatelet and anticoagulant medications, relatively little work has been reported on the natural history of ASDHs. Most published reports are based on retrospective reviews of case series or of large public registries.

The authors have nothing to disclose.
Department of Neurosurgery, Virginia Commonwealth University, 417 North 11th Street, 6th Floor, PO Box 980631, Richmond, VA 23298-0631, USA
* Corresponding author.
E-mail address: avaladka@gmail.com

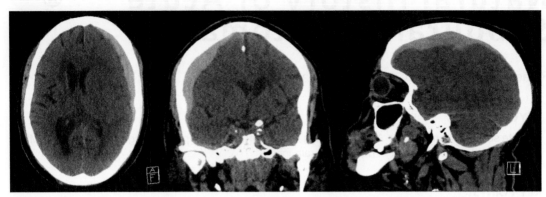

Fig. 1. Representative CT images of a left convexity ASDH with no underlying skull fracture (*axial, coronal, and sagittal, from left to right, respectively*). There is a small amount of left-to-right midline shift with mass effect on the left lateral ventricle. The basilar cisterns are preserved, without signs of herniation.

DEMOGRAPHICS

Traumatic brain injury (TBI) is a significant cause of mortality and permanent disability across the globe. TBI represents a spectrum of disease processes that ranges from concussion to large intra-axial and extra-axial intracranial hematomas, including ASDH.

For patients with TBI in general, outcomes have improved somewhat over the past decades because of better organization of emergency medical systems, greater speed and quality of computed tomography (CT) scanning, and refinements in general critical care practices.

However, mortality and outcome in patients with ASDH have not seen as much improvement. Mortality has been reported to range from 50% to 90%[1–4] or even higher in some series that include patients receiving anticoagulant therapies.[5] Associated intracranial and extracranial injuries are common and may contribute to

increased morbidity and mortality.[6] Overall outcomes may worsen in coming years as the population ages.

SPECIFIC TYPES OF ACUTE SUBDURAL HEMATOMA

The natural history of a subdural hematoma (SDH) is influenced by whether it is traumatic or nontraumatic in origin (**Table 1**). A retrospective cohort study based on several statewide administrative claims databases analyzed more than 27,000 patients with conservatively managed SDH. This study included both traumatic SDH, identified by such International Classification of Diseases, Ninth Revision, Clinical Modification (ICD-9-CM) discharge codes as 852.2x or 852.3x, and nontraumatic SDH, coded as 432.1.[7] Approximately 71% of all cases were traumatic SDHs, and 29% were nontraumatic. This latter group had higher rates of subsequent SDH-related hospitalization,

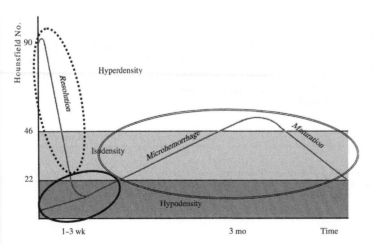

Fig. 2. Sequential change of CT density of an ASDH and its proposed mechanism. (*From* Lee KS. Natural history of chronic subdural haematoma. [Review]. Brain Injury 2004;18: 354; with permission.)

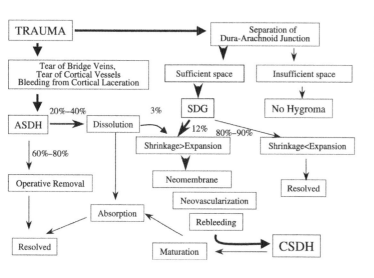

Fig. 3. Schematic representation of the origin and pathogenesis of SDHs and the relationship among the 3 traumatic subdural lesions. SDG, subdural hygroma. (*From* Lee KS. Natural history of chronic subdural haematoma. [Review]. Brain Injury 2004;18:356; with permission.)

surgery, and death. The overall readmission rate within 90 days for SDH was approximately 1 in 8.

Parafalcine and Tentorial Acute Subdural Hematoma

Certain subtypes of traumatic ASDH and certain patient characteristics taken together may portend a benign course. Howard and colleagues[8] found that isolated thin parafalcine and tentorial ASDHs in younger patients with mild TBI (Glasgow Coma Scale [GCS] score 13–15) did not enlarge, even when patients were taking antiplatelet or anticoagulant agents, or both. They suggested that such patients could be managed on a standard medical/surgical ward and did not require observation in an intensive care unit or intermediate care unit. However, only 65 patients met inclusion criteria for their study, which represented 8% of all patients admitted to their Level I trauma center with an ICD-9 code for SDH after closed head injury.

Posterior Fossa Acute Subdural Hematoma

Although rare, traumatic posterior fossa ASDHs are often associated with poor outcome. In a retrospective analysis of their experience with 10 patients, Takeuchi and colleagues[9] reported a 90% poor outcome rate and a 50% mortality rate in patients with posterior fossa ASDH. Half of their patients exhibited coagulopathy. Their review of the literature revealed that posterior fossa SDHs were associated with occipital impacts and fractures, low GCS score, additional intracranial lesions (especially supratentorial lesions and intracerebellar hematomas), a significant rate of lesion evolution within the first 2 postinjury days, and high rates of poor outcome and mortality. Similarly, Oliveira de Amorim and colleagues[10] retrospectively identified 4 cases of traumatic posterior fossa ASDH from their own institution and added an additional 57 cases from the literature. More than half the patients had an initial GCS score below 8, and unfavorable outcomes were recorded in 63%.

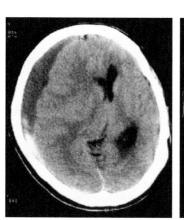 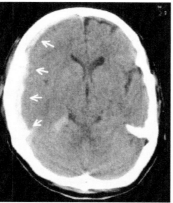

Fig. 4. The left axial CT image illustrates a CSDH. The image on the right depicts the original ASDH (*arrows*) from which the chronic hematoma originated.

Table 1
Etiologies of acute subdural hematomas

Type	Causes
Trauma	Motor vehicle collisions, falls, assaults, accidents
Coagulopathy or medical anticoagulation	Warfarin, heparin, hemophilia, liver disease, thrombocytopenia
Nontraumatic hemorrhage	Cerebral aneurysm, arteriovenous malformation, tumor (especially meningioma or dural metastasis)
Postsurgical	Craniotomy, CSF shunting
Intracranial hypotension	Lumbar puncture, lumbar CSF leak, lumboperitoneal shunt, spinal epidural anesthesia
Inflicted injury	Usually pediatric age group; also can be seen in the elderly
Spontaneous or unknown	Rare

Abbreviation: CSF, cerebrospinal fluid.

Nontraumatic Acute Subdural Hematoma

Numerous nontraumatic conditions may cause ASDH, either as a result of direct bleeding into the subdural space or as an extension of an intraparenchymal hematoma into the subdural space. These conditions include (1) ruptured intracranial aneurysm, (2) ruptured cortical artery, (3) hypertensive cerebral hemorrhage, (4) neoplasm, (5) hematologic disorder, (6) anticoagulant or thrombolytic therapy, (7) cerebral amyloid angiopathy, (8) dural arteriovenous fistula, and (9) acquired immune deficiency syndrome (**Table 2**).[11]

INITIAL DECISION-MAKING

The decision about whether to pursue nonoperative management of a patient with ASDH or to proceed with surgery is guided by the clinical examination and by imaging findings. The bedside examination can be repeated as often as desired. However, repeating imaging at frequent intervals can be unduly burdensome. It also increases costs and adds to a patient's cumulative radiation exposure. Many reports have demonstrated success in not obtaining follow-up CT scans in certain patients whose neurologic examinations remain at or near normal. This strategy is especially well-suited for patients with very small traumatic hemorrhagic lesions and clinically mild injuries. Very thin, low-volume SDHs may fall into this category.

With larger ASDHs, concern about potential enlargement may prompt follow-up CT scanning roughly 4 to 6 hours after an initial scan. Significant expansion of an ASDH may lead to immediate surgery before the patient exhibits associated clinical findings. Less dramatic growth of the lesion may lead to plans for another scan several hours later to determine if the clot has stabilized, or if it has continued to enlarge and may thus require surgical evacuation. Deciding to take a patient for surgical evacuation of an ASDH because of lesion growth on imaging studies, rather than change in neurologic examination, may occur more commonly in elderly patients. Age-associated cerebral atrophy may allow such patients to harbor relatively large hematomas without initially demonstrating symptoms. But after 1 or 2 days, edema of compressed brain tissue and of the hematoma itself may lead to neurologic worsening even if the active bleeding that created the hematoma has ceased.

Antiplatelet and Anticoagulant Medications

A patient's use of anticoagulants and/or newer antiplatelet medications would seem to be an obvious risk factor for enlargement of a small ASDH. However, some published reports fail to support this assumption or even provide data to refute it. The retrospective design of these studies and of their data collection may partially explain such findings. Aggressive reversal of these medications should be the neurosurgeon's standard approach, modified as necessary by the particular circumstances of each individual case.

Ivascu and colleagues[12] reported that even an emergency department protocol for prompt physician evaluation of patients known to be taking anticoagulant medications does not improve outcomes without a concomitant protocol for aggressive therapeutic intervention. The generalizability of these results may be limited because types of intracranial hemorrhage other than ASDH also were included, and more importantly, many anticoagulants other than warfarin are now in widespread use. Reversal of these other agents is very difficult or even not possible in some cases. But the underlying message that speedy treatment is essential is one that should be remembered by emergency physicians and others who see these patients soon after trauma.

The influence of anticoagulant or antiplatelet medications in the transformation of a small ASDH into a CSDH that is large enough to require

Table 2
Nontraumatic causes of acute subdural hematomas

Type	Epidemiology	Brief Discussion
Ruptured intracranial aneurysm	2%–10% of ruptured aneurysms result in SDH. Typically women.	In most cases there is an associated subarachnoid hemorrhage. The location of the responsible aneurysm is most often the internal carotid artery or the anterior communicating artery.
Ruptured cortical artery	Spontaneous rupture occurs predominantly in men. Accounts for 80% of reported cases.	The location in all cases reported is typically a vessel at or near the Sylvian fissure, originating from branches of the middle cerebral artery. The anatomic arrangement that predisposes to spontaneous rupture includes a fragile right-angled artery or an artery "bridging" the subdural space.
Hypertensive intracerebral hemorrhage	Reported to occur in 6% of hypertensive hemorrhages and most often involves cerebellar hematomas.	SDH may result from extension of an intracerebral hypertensive hemorrhage rupturing through the cerebral cortex to involve the subdural space. Hypertension may also result in SDH by causing rupture of a cortical artery.
Neoplasm	Most common malignancies associated with SDH are leukemia and metastatic carcinoma.	A variety of neoplasms are associated with SDH. These include primary tumors of the brain and its coverings, hematologic malignancies, and metastatic tumors. In some cases, SDH may be the first symptoms of the tumor.
Hematological disorder	Typical age of the individual is <18 y, but may also occur in neonates and infants.	In most cases of disorders of the hematopoietic system, factor deficiency (inherited or acquired) is the most common type. Individuals with Factor VIII and IX deficiency have factor activity levels of 0–1 U/dL. Fatal nontraumatic SDH has been reported in an individual with lupus anticoagulant.
Other conditions	—	Nontraumatic SDH has been described in conditions that include therapy with anticoagulants, thrombolytic therapy, cerebral amyloid angiopathy, dural arteriovenous fistulas, and acquired immune deficiency syndrome.

Abbreviation: SDH, subdural hematoma.

surgical drainage is unclear. It is possible that any such effect varies both with the specific medication and/or also with the dosage. Laviv and Rappaport[13] retrospectively analyzed their experience with conservative management of patients with ASDH. They reported that, of 21 patients taking anticoagulants, antiaggregants, or clopidogrel, 20 (95%) later underwent surgical drainage of a CSDH. Overall, the group that developed surgically treated CSDHs had thicker initial hematomas than the nonoperated group.[13]

NONOPERATIVE MANAGEMENT

Significant medical comorbidities are common in elderly patients and are often of sufficient severity to preclude an intervention as aggressive as a craniotomy. The cerebral atrophy that accompanies normal aging offers some protection from ASDH by creating extra intracranial volume into which an acute hematoma can expand, thus allowing nonoperative management to be successful in many cases.

The greatest risk of nonoperative management is the potential for neurologic deterioration. This risk, and the likelihood of subsequent permanent neurologic impairment, must be considered in the context of the risks of surgical intervention. There appears to be little acute risk of other complications of nonoperative management of these patients. Seizures have not been reported to occur more commonly in patients with an unevacuated ASDH. The same is true regarding ischemic injury to compressed underlying brain tissue.

A related question is the setting in which such patients should be observed. There are at least 2 factors that must be considered.

- The first is early detection of neurologic deterioration. Because of the need to detect such an event quickly and then to initiate immediate action, many patients are better off in an intensive care unit or similar setting in which they can be assessed frequently by trained examiners.
- The other factor is prompt access to neurosurgical intervention. Securing prompt access does not necessarily require that all such patients must be physically transferred to a hospital with around-the-clock access to a neurosurgical operating room. If foolproof mechanisms have been created for immediate transfer of worsening patients to a neurosurgical facility, then observation at the original hospital may be reasonable in many cases because relatively few such patients will suffer neurologic deterioration.

Progression to Chronic Subdural Hematoma After Conservative Management

Occasionally, patients with large ASDHs who would normally be taken for surgical evacuation may be too frail or may have such significant underlying comorbidities that subjecting them to general anesthesia and craniotomy is not a viable option, even if they display unilateral weakness or other signs of mass effect. Allowing several days to pass so that the solid acute hematoma undergoes significant liquefaction as it progresses to a subacute hematoma may be the best approach in some of these cases because the liquefied hematoma often can be drained through a bur hole or other minimally invasive approach under local anesthesia.

In a retrospectively analyzed series of 177 patients, Lee and colleagues[14] compared 16 patients (9%) in whom nonoperatively managed ASDH progressed to CSDH requiring surgical evacuation with 161 patients in whom ASDH resolved with conservative management. These investigators found that older age and larger hematoma size were associated with progression of ASDH to symptomatic CSDH. They also found a slightly higher hematoma density as measured in Hounsfield units. They did not find a correlation with use of anticoagulant or antiplatelet agents, but the numbers of such patients were small, and abnormal clotting parameters were treated with blood products, thus obscuring any potential effect of these medications.

In another series of 27 patients with traumatic ASDH who were managed nonoperatively, 1 (4%) deteriorated and required craniotomy.[15] Four patients (15%) demonstrated evolution into CSDH and underwent bur hole drainage 15 to 21 days after injury. The remaining 22 patients (81%) required no additional treatment. No patients developed seizures. Mean duration of follow-up was 6 weeks.

Spontaneous Resolution of Acute Subdural Hematoma

Case reports stretching back over decades have documented apparent resolution of ASDHs in patients with obvious neurologic compromise from the hematomas, including coma, asymmetric motor findings, and unilateral pupillary dilatation. Concurrent injuries, underlying medical comorbidities, and/or family refusal to consent to surgery represent reasons why emergency craniotomy was not performed.

Wen and colleagues[16] described their experience with such a patient and identified 19 additional cases in the literature. They reported that the following features seem to characterize most of these cases: (1) coma less than 12 hours in duration after the initial injury; (2) absence of cerebral contusion; (3) thin width and wide distribution of the hematoma; (4) presence of a low-density band between the hematoma and the inner table of the skull on initial CT scan; and (5) lack of severe initial TBI, with initial GCS score greater than 8.

Fujimoto and colleagues[17] retrospectively reviewed 56 patients with ASDH with midline shift of more than 10 mm and clot thickness larger than 10 mm who did not undergo immediate surgery, most commonly because of advanced age, poor general condition, or family wishes, or because patients did not exhibit significant neurologic symptoms. Rapid spontaneous resolution of the ASDH was defined as neurologic improvement within 24 hours and decrease of hematoma thickness by more than 5 mm within 96 hours. Eighteen patients (32%) demonstrated rapid spontaneous resolution. Multivariate analysis found that preinjury use of antiplatelet agents and presence of a low-density band between the hematoma and the inner wall of the skull on initial CT scan were independent predictive factors for rapid spontaneous resolution.

Commonly proposed explanations for rapid decrease in size and mass effect of an ASDH include a tear in the arachnoid that permits cerebrospinal fluid to wash away the acute blood, and/or redistribution rather than true resorption of the acute blood, which may be facilitated by a decrease in intracranial pressure after treating physicians' medical interventions. Interestingly, however, others have reported that decreasing brain compliance by adjusting upward the valve setting of an already-present ventriculoperitoneal shunt was associated with disappearance of an ASDH within 6 days.[18] Of course, the very fact that these cases are unusual enough to merit publication demonstrates how rare it is for a sizable ASDH to resolve rapidly. Immediate surgery is the recommended treatment for these patients.

OUTCOMES WITH NONOPERATIVE MANAGEMENT

Acute deterioration has been recognized for decades as a potential outcome of nonoperative management of patients with acute traumatic intracranial hemorrhage. The terms "talk and deteriorate" or "talk and die" vividly describe this phenomenon. In 1987, Rockswold and colleagues[19] reported on 33 of 215 patients with severe TBI who exhibited such deterioration. Twenty-five (76%) of these 33 patients underwent surgery, and of those 25, 14 had ASDHs. More aggressive

use of early follow-up CT scanning in recent years seems to have lowered the rate of such events, but they still occur with sufficient frequency that virtually every neurosurgeon has personal experience with this type of patient.

In a 1994 review at their Level I trauma center of ASDH management in 83 patients with GCS score 11 to 15, Croce and colleagues[20] found that nonoperatively managed patients had fewer focal neurologic deficits, smaller hematomas, and less cisternal effacement. Outcomes did not differ between groups. Of the 58 patients managed nonsurgically, 6% later required surgery for CSDH.

Bullock and colleagues attempted nonoperative management in 23 conscious patients (3%) of 837 with traumatic ASDH.[2] In a retrospective analysis, they report that 6 (26%) of the 23 later underwent burr hole drainage of their hematomas at a mean of 15 days after injury. The ASDHs in the 6 operated patients were significantly larger than in the other 17 patients. The investigators proposed the following criteria for attempting nonoperative management of patients with traumatic ASDH: (1) GCS score greater than or equal to 13; (2) absence of associated intraparenchymal hematomas, contusions, or edema; (3) midline shift less than 10 mm; and (4) absence of basal cisternal effacement.

Ellenbogen and colleagues reviewed outcomes in 1427 patients with ASDH referred to their Level I trauma center. Such a population would be expected to have an overall greater severity of injury than that seen at most hospitals. GCS score exceeded 12 in only 58% of patients. Mean age was 58 years. A total of 248 (17%) patients underwent surgical evacuation of their SDHs. Mean length of stay was 9.6 days, and 40% spent 2 or more days in the intensive care unit. Overall inpatient mortality was 16% and was essentially the same in operated and nonoperated groups. Medical complications occurred in 28% of the overall series and most commonly consisted of pneumonia, urinary tract infection, or acute respiratory distress syndrome. Complications did not differ between operated and nonoperated patients. At discharge, 94% of patients had a GCS score of more than 12. The investigators note that their mortality rate was lower than that reported in other studies of traumatic ASDH and that their rates of deep venous thrombosis and pulmonary embolism were lower than expected. They suggest that earlier diagnosis of ASDH and improvement in care from regionalization of emergency medical systems may explain their findings.[21]

Kim and colleagues[22] described 98 patients with mild TBI (GCS score 13–15) and ASDH in whom outcome was assessed by enlargement of the SDH on subsequent imaging and by the need for subsequent surgical evacuation. Roughly two-thirds of these patients demonstrated regression of the SDH. The other 35% underwent delayed surgical evacuation at a median of 17 days after injury. Larger hematoma volume and midline shift were associated with the need for delayed hematoma evacuation. Interestingly, subarachnoid hemorrhage and cerebral contusions were more common in the nonoperative group. Reasons for the higher failure rate of conservative management in this series as compared with those in other reports are unclear and may relate to a lower threshold for taking patients to the operating room for delayed evacuation of an SDH.

Feliciano and colleagues[23] reported outcomes of nonoperated ASDH in a series of 38 patients, roughly half of whom were younger than 65 years. In 87% of these patients, midline shift was 5 mm or less, and hematoma thickness was 10 mm or less. Six patients in this group were taking antiplatelet or anticoagulant medications, and some were treated with blood products. Use of these medications was not associated with outcome in this subgroup with smaller hematomas. None of these patients required surgery. In the other 5 patients with hematoma thickness of more than 10 mm or shift greater than 5 mm, surgery was not performed because of excessive cardiac risk or withholding of consent by relatives. One patient in this group required surgery for neurologic deterioration.

Bajsarowicz and colleagues[24] retrospectively reviewed 646 patients with traumatic ASDH who were initially treated conservatively. Forty-two patients eventually required delayed surgical intervention after a median of 9.5 days, most commonly for symptomatic enlargement of the hematoma (median 14 days) or development of increased intracranial pressure (median 3.5 days). Factors associated with deterioration were thicker SDH, greater midline shift, location at the cerebral convexity, history of falls, and alcohol abuse.

SUMMARY

Published literature and widespread clinical experience make it clear that most ASDHs can be managed nonoperatively. This is especially true for smaller lesions in patients with good neurologic status. Even in patients who present with severe neurologic deficits or coma, the benefit of evacuating small ASDHs is often unclear. These ASDHs usually resolve spontaneously.

Large ASDHs may require a different approach. When a comatose patient is found to have a large ASDH associated with compression of the basal cisterns, significant midline shift, or other signs of mass effect, immediate surgery is the default management plan.

More problematic is the management of large ASDHs in patients with no or minimal symptoms. Conservative management may be considered in patients in good neurologic status and, despite the size of the ASDH, relatively little underlying mass effect.

The effect of anticoagulant and antiplatelet medications on the natural history of ASDH is not clear from the literature. Prudence would suggest that reversal of such agents be considered in all patients with ASDH. Likewise, a lower threshold for early repeat CT scanning may be appropriate in patients with ASDH who are taking such medications.

Even if nonoperative management is successful in the acute phase, the risk remains for subsequent progression of an ASDH into a CSDH that is large enough to require surgery. Again, the literature is unclear on the effects of anticoagulants or antihypertensives on such a progression. Scheduled CT scanning 1 to 2 weeks after development of an ASDH may detect this process before clinical symptoms appear.

REFERENCES

1. Massaro F, Lanotte M, Faccani G, et al. One hundred and twenty-seven cases of acute subdural haematoma operated on. Acta Neurochir (Wien) 1996;138:185–91.
2. Mathew P, Oluoch-Olunya DL, Condon BR, et al. Acute subdural haematoma in the conscious patient: outcome with initial non-operative management. Acta Neurochir (Wien) 1993;121:100–8.
3. Seelig JM, Becker DP, Miller JD, et al. Traumatic acute subdural hematoma: major mortality reduction in comatose patients treated within four hours. N Engl J Med 1981;304:1511–8.
4. Zumkeller M, Behrmann R, Heissler HE, et al. Computed tomographic criteria and survival rate for patients with acute subdural hematoma. Neurosurgery 1996;39:708–13.
5. Kawamata T, Takeshita M, Kubo O, et al. Management of intracranial hemorrhage associated with anticoagulant therapy. Surg Neurol 1995;44:438–43.
6. Bullock MR, Chesnut R, Ghajar J, et al. Surgical management of acute subdural hematomas. Neurosurgery 2006;58(3 Suppl):S16–24.
7. Morris NA, Merkler AE, Parker WE, et al. Adverse outcomes after initial non-surgical management of subdural hematoma: a population-based study. Neurocrit Care 2016;24:226–32.
8. Howard BM, Rindler RS, Holland CM, et al. Management and outcomes of isolated tentorial and parafalcine "smear" subdural hematomas at a level-1

trauma center: necessity of high acuity care. J Neurotrauma 2016. [Epub ahead of print].

9. Takeuchi S, Takasato Y, Wada K, et al. Traumatic posterior fossa subdural hematomas. J Trauma Acute Care Surg 2012;72:480–6.

10. de Amorim RLO, Stiver SI, Paiva WS, et al. Treatment of traumatic acute posterior fossa subdural hematoma: report of four cases with systematic review and management algorithm. Acta Neurochir (Wien) 2014;156:199–206.

11. Avis SP. Nontraumatic acute subdural hematoma. A case report and review of the literature. Am J Forensic Med Pathol 1993;14:130–4.

12. Ivascu FA, Janczyk RJ, Junn FS, et al. Treatment of trauma patients with intracranial hemorrhage on pre-injury warfarin. J Trauma 2006;61:318–21.

13. Laviv Y, Rappaport ZH. Risk factors for development of significant chronic subdural hematoma following conservative treatment of acute subdural hemorrhage. Br J Neurosurg 2014;28:733–8.

14. Lee JJ, Won Y, Yang T, et al. Risk factors of chronic subdural hematoma progression after conservative management of cases with initially acute subdural hematoma. Korean J Neurotrauma 2015;11:52–7.

15. Ahmed E, Aurangzeb A, Khan SA, et al. Frequency of conservatively managed traumatic acute subdural haematoma changing into chronic subdural haematoma. J Ayub Med Coll Abbottabad 2012;24:71–4.

16. Wen L, Liu WG, Ma L, et al. Spontaneous rapid resolution of acute subdural hematoma after head trauma: is it truly rare? Case report and relevant review of the literature. Ir J Med Sci 2009;178:367–71.

17. Fujimoto K, Otsuka T, Yoshizato K, et al. Predictors of rapid spontaneous resolution of acute subdural hematoma. Clin Neurol Neurosurg 2014;118:94–7.

18. Hayes J, Roguski M, Riesenburger RI. Rapid resolution of an acute subdural hematoma by increasing the shunt valve pressure in a 63-year-old man with normal-pressure hydrocephalus with a ventriculo-peritoneal shunt: a case report and literature review. J Med Case Rep 2012;6:393.

19. Rockswold GR, Leonard PR, Nagib MG. Analysis of management in thirty-three closed head injury patients who "talked and deteriorated". Neurosurgery 1987;21:51–5.

20. Croce MA, Dent DL, Menke PG, et al. Acute subdural hematoma: nonsurgical management of selected patients. J Trauma 1994;36:820–7.

21. Ryan CG, Thompson RE, Temkin NR, et al. Acute traumatic subdural hematoma: current mortality and functional outcomes in adult patients at a Level I trauma center. J Trauma Acute Care Surg 2012;73:1348–54.

22. Kim BJ, Park KJ, Park DH, et al. Risk factors of delayed surgical evacuation for initially nonoperative acute subdural hematomas following mild head injury. Acta Neurochir (Wien) 2014;156:1605–13.

23. Feliciano CE, De Jesús O. Conservative management outcomes of traumatic acute subdural hematomas. P R Health Sci J 2008;27:220–3.

24. Bajsarowicz P, Prakash I, Lamoureux J, et al. Nonsurgical acute traumatic subdural hematoma: what is the risk? J Neurosurg 2015;123:1176–83.

Cranioplasty

Matthew Piazza, MD, M. Sean Grady, MD*

KEYWORDS

- Cranioplasty • Autologous cranioplasty • Synthetic cranioplasty • Skull reconstruction
- Cranial defect • Methyl methacrylate

KEY POINTS

- Cranioplasty restores the normal cranial architecture and protective functions of the skull and may play a role in normalizing cerebrospinal fluid dynamics in patients undergoing large craniectomies for trauma.
- The ideal material for cranioplasty is lightweight, durable, easily fixable to the skull, osteoconductive, and malleable.
- Separation of the scalp flap and temporalis muscle from the underlying dura or dural substitute is critical for a good outcome.
- Cranioplasty, like any neurosurgical procedure, has specific complications with which neurosurgeons must be familiar.

INTRODUCTION

Skull defects and craniofacial bone abnormalities that require reconstruction are common in a variety of neurosurgical procedures. From the patient's perspective, the primary reason for repair of these defects may be cosmetic. However, cranial bone provides important support and restores normal cerebrospinal fluid (CSF) flow dynamics, reducing the formation of pseudomeningoceles and protecting vital structures. Craniofacial reconstruction and cranioplasty have a long history, but new surgical techniques and a multitude of material options have recently fueled advancement in this area. This article describes the clinical indications for cranioplasty, preoperative management and timing of reconstruction, materials, and operative techniques.

CLINICAL INDICATIONS FOR CRANIOPLASTY

Although largely an elective procedure, cranioplasty has several important indications and can improve quality of life for postcraniectomy patients. Following craniectomy, patients can develop skin depression and a sunken flap that can lead to an asymmetric appearance of the head. Although seemingly innocuous, this abnormal appearance can have major negative implications on the psychological well-being of the patient as well as how the patient is perceived by other people. Restoring the normal architecture of the skull can have significant psychosocial benefits to the patient as well as reestablishing the protective barrier of the skull.

Craniectomy essentially nullifies the Monroe-Kellie doctrine that governs intracranial pressure, CSF dynamics, and ultimately cerebral blood flow and can give rise to several complications, including extra-axial fluid collections; hydrocephalus; and sunken flap syndrome, also known as syndrome of the trephined. Sunken flap syndrome results from a combination of receding brain as swelling resolves, disturbances in CSF dynamics, and effects of atmospheric pressure.

Disclosure: The authors have nothing to disclose.
Article reprinted from Piazza MA, Grady MS. Cranioplasty. In: Winn HR, ed. Youmans and Winn Neurological Surgery. 7th ed. Philadelphia: Elsevier; 2017:280, e150–e156 with permission from Elsevier.
Department of Neurosurgery, Hospital of the University of Pennsylvania, 3400 Spruce Street, 3rd Floor Silverstein, Philadelphia, PA 19104, USA
* Corresponding author.
E-mail address: Michael.grady@uphs.upenn.edu

Neurosurg Clin N Am 28 (2017) 257–265
http://dx.doi.org/10.1016/j.nec.2016.11.008
1042-3680/17/© 2016 Elsevier Inc. All rights reserved.

Miscellaneous neurologic symptoms are attributed to the hemispheric collapse and include headache, dizziness, fatigue, and psychiatric changes.[1] Replacement of bone flap has been shown to lead to neurologic improvement, mostly in motor function, in small case series.[2] Transcranial Doppler ultrasonography has shown improvement in cerebral blood flow following cranioplasty.[3] Larger, controlled studies are needed to better understand the relationship between cranioplasty, cerebral hemodynamics, and clinical outcome.

TIMING OF CRANIOPLASTY

Timing of cranioplasty depends largely on the indication for craniectomy. Immediate cranioplasty has rare indications and may be performed for craniectomy for neoplastic invasion of cranium. Delayed cranioplasty is usually indicated for removal of bone flap for intracranial infection or medically refractory intracranial hypertension.

In cases of intracranial infection with suspected involvement and devitalization of bone, craniectomy is commonly performed. Although recent, small case series have shown the feasibility and safety of immediate titanium cranioplasty after bone flap infection,[4] usually time intervals between craniectomy and cranioplasty between 6 weeks and 1 year have been identified.[5] Ultimately the timing of cranioplasty is patient tailored and sufficient time must pass for adequate treatment and clearance of cranial (as well as any systemic) infection. The previous incision must be well healed and surrounding tissues must be vascularized. Inflammatory markers, such as C-reactive protein and erythrocyte sedimentation rate, as well as serial imaging, may assist in the determination of cranioplasty timing.

In patients who undergo decompressive craniectomy for intracranial hypertension (**Fig. 1**) in the setting of traumatic brain injury or stroke, the patient's neurologic status and intracranial pressure must have stabilized and the patient should be free of both systemic and cranial infection. As in cases of cranioplasty after intracranial infection, the patient's incision should be healed completely. Traditionally, cranioplasty after decompressive craniectomy is performed at approximately 3 months, allowing sufficient time for neurologic and medical recovery, but the optimal timing remains controversial. Some practitioners have argued that early cranioplasty may improve CSF dynamics and lead to better neurologic recovery, although conflicting data in the literature suggest that larger prospective studies of the relationship between timing of cranioplasty and neurologic outcome are needed.[6–9]

On a technical note, early cranioplasty after 5 to 8 weeks may allow easier discrimination of the various tissue layers when the skin flap is reflected. However, onlay synthetic dural substitutes, if used, may not have formed an adherence to the underlying native dura and are often inadvertently reflected with the skin flap.

PREOPERATIVE MANAGEMENT

Once the decision to perform cranioplasty is made, important preoperative studies include computed tomography with bone windows; three-dimensional reconstruction may further guide operative management. MRI is occasionally useful if there is a question about the relation of soft tissue structures, such as scalp or dura, to the skull defect. In addition, preoperative management must include a thorough investigation of the patient's underlying health status and search for

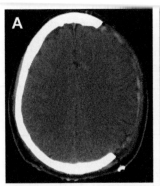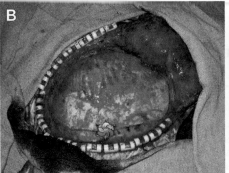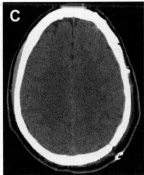

Fig. 1. Cranioplasty after left decompressive hemicraniectomy for intractable intracranial hypertension. (*A*) Preoperative computed tomographic scan showing left skull defect. (*B*) Intraoperative view of autologous bone flap secured to native skull with plating system. (*C*) Postoperative computed tomographic scan showing cranioplasty. (*From* Piazza M, Sean Grady M. Cranioplasty. In: Winn HR, ed. Youmans and Winn neurologic surgery. 7th edition. Philadelphia: Elsevier, 2017; with permission.)

any contraindications to cranioplasty. Patients who are hemodynamically unstable, are bacteremic, or have persistent intracranial hypertension may be deferred until a later time. In our practice, we defer cranioplasty if the patient has any active infection, including Clostridium difficile. Although it is unlikely that a gastrointestinal infection would contaminate the cranioplasty, this scenario is difficult to rule out when the patient is postoperative and actively febrile. In general, cranioplasty is an elective procedure and should be undertaken only when these other medical issues have resolved.

In cases of traumatic brain injury or stroke, the patient's autologous bone flap must be removed from storage before cranioplasty. Autologous bone flaps are usually either placed into deep-freeze preservation or subcutaneously preserved in abdominal fat. Some reports indicate that the preservation in subcutaneous tissue improves the bone viability, thereby lowering cranioplasty revision rate.[10] However, storage at less than −28°C has been shown to be an effective method of preservation and avoids the additional morbidity of an abdominal incision.[11–14] The largest disadvantage of frozen autologous bone graft is a higher rate of reported resorption compared with other cranioplasty materials, especially in children.[15,16] Autologous bone flaps placed in deep-freeze preservation may be removed from storage on the morning of surgery.

Infection of the autologous bone flap is also a common complication, and sterile technique and care must be taken during the collection and storage preservation of the bone flap at the time of hemicraniectomy. Use of ethylene oxide gas to sterilize autologous bone graft before storage at room temperature has been shown to be an effective alternative to freezing the bone flap.[17] Cultures of the bone flap obtained at this time must be reviewed before cranioplasty, because bacterial contamination of the bone flap often occurs in an indolent fashion.[18] The most common isolated organisms are Propionibacterium acnes, Staphylococcus aureus, and coagulase-negative Staphylococcus. Traditionally, bacterial contamination of an autologous bone flap has been a contraindication for reinsertion during cranioplasty, although recent literation suggests that reimplanting bone flaps with positive culture swabs does not increase the risk of postoperative infection.[19]

CRANIOPLASTY MATERIAL OPTIONS

There is a large selection of possible materials for repair of skull defects, which may be categorized into autografts, allografts, xenografts, and bone substitutes. The success and durability of the operation require careful selection of a material tailored to the clinical scenario. The ideal material is malleable, sterilizable, nonmagnetic, radiolucent, lightweight, and able to be easily secured to existing skull (**Table 1**).

Methyl methacrylate is polymerized ester of acrylic acid that exists in powdered form and is mixed with a liquid monomer, benzoyl peroxide. In an exothermic reaction, methyl methacrylate slowly cools from a pastelike substance into a translucent material with strength comparable with that of native bone.[20] During this cooling phase, methyl methacrylate may be shaped to fit any skull defect. Methyl methacrylate may be used for technically challenging areas of the skull, and reconstruction and growth from the native bone edge adjacent to the prosthesis secures it to the skull. Disadvantages of methyl methacrylate include postoperative infection, at a rate of approximately 5% to 10%, and plate breakdown or fracture.[21,22] A methyl methacrylate prosthesis is at higher risk of infection compared with autologous bone flap because it is not viable, and a fibrous layer grows around the plate, to which bacteria may adhere. The most common organisms are S aureus and P acnes.[23] Deep wound infection may be latent and not become clinically apparent for several years. Liquid methyl methacrylate may be absorbed by tissues and has been reported to cause acute hypotension and hypersensitivity.[24,25] Different types of methyl methacrylate are commercially available. It is a composite material of polymethyl methacrylate and barium sulfate, creating a radiopaque bone cement.

Another option of synthetic prostheses is calcium phosphate bone cement, which, like methyl methacrylate, exists as a powder and forms a malleable substance when it is mixed with liquid sodium phosphate. When it is fully cured, the calcium phosphate prosthesis approximates the mineral phase of bone and is integrated into the native skull and remodeled over time to fit the defect. The most commonly used calcium phosphate material is hydroxyapatite, shown to be ideally suited for small craniofacial defects.[26,27] When it is used directly against exposed dura, titanium mesh is recommended as an underlay to prevent small fractures in the hydroxyapatite plate from dural pulsations.[28] In contrast with methyl methacrylate, which does not allow further expansion of a growing skull, hydroxyapatite bone cement is often used for skull defects in the pediatric population. Certain types of calcium phosphate prostheses, including hydroxyapatite, have the additional advantage of being osteoconductive,

Table 1
Comparison of cranioplasty materials

Material	Implant Type	Advantages	Disadvantages
Autologous bone	Autograft	Viable, potential for growth, low rate of plate fracture or migration	Bone resorption, infection, possible poor cosmesis
Titanium mesh	Metal	No inflammatory reaction, low infection rate, osteointegrative	High cost, poor malleability, possible poor cosmesis, loosens over time; image artifact on magnetic resonance images and computed tomographic scans, rendering resolution of adjacent tissue difficult
Porous polyethylene implants	Polymer	Osseous and fibrovascular ingrowth, minimal imaging artifact, low infection rate	Removal may be difficult because of native tissue ingrowth
Methyl methacrylate	Polymer	Ease of use, excellent cosmesis, low cost, strength and durability	Infection, plate fracture, no growth potential, exothermic reaction, inflammatory reaction
Calcium phosphate bone cement	Ceramic	Osteoconductive, osteoinductive, useful for difficult-to-reach defects, no inflammatory reaction	Brittle, fragile, difficult to contour, cannot bear stress
Hydroxyapatite–polymethyl methacrylate composite	Ceramic/polymer hybrid	Good osteoconductivity along the surface that does not penetrate centrally, reduced fragility	Limited clinical data

From Piazza MA, Grady MS. Cranioplasty. In: Winn HR, editor. Youmans and Winn Neurological Surgery. 7th edition. Philadelphia: Elsevier; 2017:e151 with permission from Elsevier.

so they serve as scaffolding for growth of new bone.

Titanium mesh, either alone or in combination with methyl methacrylate, is another useful material for cranioplasty. Titanium is nonferromagnetic and noncorrosive, and it does not elicit an inflammatory reaction. Several series have reported a low incidence of infection while still achieving excellent cosmetic results.[29,30] Most commonly, titanium exists as a metallic alloy with other metals to improve its strength and malleability. Titanium is also used to preform prostheses using three-dimensional computed tomographic reconstructions of the skull base defect.

Computer-designed implants from computed tomographic reconstructions are expensive but effective for complex skull defects.[31] Anatomic models may be formed by polymerization of ultraviolet light–sensitive liquid resin with use of a laser, based on computed tomographic data. These stereolithographic models are then used to manufacture customized titanium plates, hydroxyapatite implants, or methyl methacrylate prostheses.[32] Costs for these prefabricated prostheses

may be as high as $4000; however, the precision has been reported to be 0.25 mm for implants as large as 18 cm.[33]

New biocompatible materials and composite implants have recently been used for cranioplasty with excellent results. Porous polyethylene implants are composed of high-density polyethylene microspheres that create interconnected pores, allowing ingrowth of native bone. This unique implant structure rapidly incorporates fibrovascular tissue from the patient and decreases the infection rate of the implant. Porous polyethylene implants may be shaped to cover a large variety of skull defects and secured with titanium screws to native bone. A distinct advantage of this material compared with titanium is that it does not produce artifact on postoperative computed tomographic scans and magnetic resonance images. In a study of 611 cranioplasty procedures using porous polyethylene, all patients achieved excellent cosmetic results with no postoperative infections.[34]

Further efforts to decrease cranioplasty implant infection rates have focused on antibiotic elution from hydroxyapatite cement materials.

Hydroxyapatite cement is able to be impregnated with a variety of antibiotics intraoperatively. Tobramycin, a broad-spectrum aminoglycoside with activity against *S aureus*, gram-negative bacteria, and gentamicin-resistant pseudomonal species, has shown promise in cranioplasty materials. Studies have shown a predictable concentration and sustained release of tobramycin from hydroxyapatite cement for approximately 10 days.[35]

Because each cranioplasty material has its own advantages and disadvantages, studies have examined hydroxyapatite–polymethyl methacrylate composites. Hydroxyapatite has good osteoconductivity but is fragile and cracks easily. In contrast, methyl methacrylate is easier to shape and is stronger, but it has relatively poor osteoconductivity. A composite of both materials using two-thirds hydroxyapatite and one-third methyl methacrylate showed almost the same osteoconductivity as hydroxyapatite alone at the surface of the implant, but it did not penetrate inside the composite.[36] Various formulas of composites show excellent promise in cranioplasty because of the different properties of each substance.

OPERATIVE TECHNIQUE

Preoperative antibiotics are administered, and the patient is usually positioned on a foam donut or horseshoe head holder. The incision follows the prior incision, with care taken to stay directly on the scar to avoid necrosis of scalp. Blood loss in these operations may be significant because of the neovascularization of scar tissue that is reincised, and it is important to alert the anesthesiologist of this possibility.

Reflection of the scalp flap is often difficult because the normal tissue planes are usually distorted. Great care should be taken to identify the plane between the galea and dura mater. A periosteal elevator or Bovie may be used to dissect these layers carefully during the reflection of the scalp. In addition, particular care must be taken in the area of the temporalis muscle because the entirety of the muscle should be reflected with the scalp flap. Failure to reflect the temporalis muscle, either independently or with the scalp, results in a suboptimal cosmetic result.

When the entirety of the skull defect is exposed and the edges of bone are clean of remaining soft tissue, the cranioplasty flap may be either fashioned or replaced if it is autologous. The key technical difference in the exposure during autologous cranioplasty is that the dura must be freed from the inner table of the native skull. Failure to do so prevents the bone flap from sitting correctly within the defect. In contrast, when methyl methacrylate is used, exposure of the outer cortex only is preferred, because it allows a thinner cranioplasty to be used and helps with proper contouring.

Occasionally, the patient's brain may have persistent herniation through the cranial defect either caused by hydrocephalus or cerebral edema precluding safe and successful replacement of the bone flap or cranial prosthesis; in this case, a brain cannula can be inserted into the lateral ventricle to drain the CSF. Thinning of the bone flap with a high-speed drill may facilitate replacement as well, although this measure may increase the risk of bone resorption. In addition, if replacement of the bone flap fails despite the measures discussed earlier, an external ventricular drain on the contralateral side or lumbar drain may be placed, CSF may be drained over the course of several days, and cranioplasty can be reattempted if swelling improves. Such patients may require a ventriculoperitoneal shunt at the time of cranioplasty, although this carries greater morbidity then when cranioplasty is performed alone.

In formation of the methyl methacrylate prosthesis, shaping of the plate to achieve an excellent cosmetic result requires careful planning. Large saline-soaked cotton balls are placed into the skull defect above the dura and molded until they form the appropriate contour (**Fig. 2**). With use of a container hooked to a vacuum system to remove fumes, the powdered methyl methacrylate and benzoyl peroxide are mixed slowly, with care taken to stir slowly so that air bubbles do not form. When the mixture reaches a thick syrup consistency, it is placed into a sterile plastic sleeve and quickly smoothed into a thin sheet. The entire plastic sleeve is placed over the skull defect, pulled taut, and pressed firmly onto the edge of the native skull. Methyl methacrylate undergoes the exothermic reaction; however, the saline-soaked cotton balls protect the underlying cortex. When the edges of the plate become more transparent, the methyl methacrylate prosthesis should be removed from the plastic sleeve and soaked briefly in cold saline. Excess acrylic may be shaved off with a high-speed drill (**Fig. 3**).

At this point, the cotton balls are removed, and the autologous bone graft or synthetic prosthesis is secured to the native skull with standard titanium plates and screws. In some situations, a central dural tack-up or dural drain may be necessary to prevent formation of postoperative epidural fluid collection. Dural tack-up sutures around the edges of the skull defect may also help prevent epidural hematomas, although the evidence for this is anecdotal. In addition, small perforations in either the autologous bone graft or methyl methacrylate plate can help prevent formation of a fluid collection

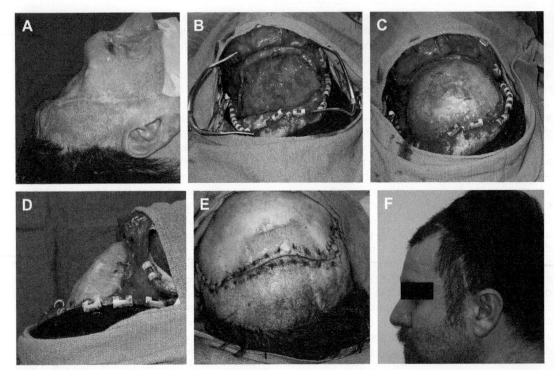

Fig. 2. Cranioplasty of bifrontal decompressive craniectomy. (*A*) Intraoperative view of skull defect. (*B*) Intraoperative view of skull defect exposure. (*C*) Methyl methacrylate plated into skull defect. (*D*) Profile view of methyl methacrylate contour. (*E*) Scalp closure and cosmetic result. (*F*) Patient at 6-week follow-up. (*From* Piazza M, Sean Grady M. Cranioplasty. In: Winn HR, ed. Youmans and Winn neurologic surgery. 7th edition. Philadelphia: Elsevier, 2017; with permission.)

beneath the prosthesis. Once the graft or implant is secured, the soft tissue layers are closed. Because the temporalis muscle is reflected with the scalp flap, it often does not need to be separated and secured to the skull. If it is raised separately, it can be attached directly to the methyl methacrylate plate by screws to act as anchor points. In the case of trauma, significant temporalis muscle wasting has often already occurred, so a perfect cosmetic result is difficult to achieve. In some cases, the scalp has retracted, and closure of the skin edges over the new bone requires careful placement of galeal sutures and vertical mattress sutures to reapproximate the scalp.

Use of a subgaleal drain is recommended after both methyl methacrylate and autologous

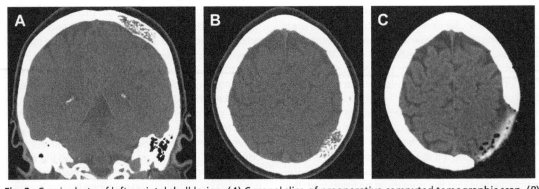

Fig. 3. Cranioplasty of left parietal skull lesion. (*A*) Coronal slice of preoperative computed tomographic scan. (*B*) Axial slice of preoperative computed tomographic scan. (*C*) Postoperative computed tomographic scan. (*From* Piazza M, Sean Grady M. Cranioplasty. In: Winn HR, ed. Youmans and Winn neurologic surgery. 7th edition. Philadelphia: Elsevier, 2017; with permission.)

cranioplasty because it prevents the extensive facial swelling that may occur after these operations. In addition, a firm and secure head wrap dressing may also assist with control of scalp edema.

POSTOPERATIVE CARE

There are different standards of practice in postoperative management of cranioplasty patients. Some surgeons routinely place patients in an intensive care setting for at least 1 night to monitor neurologic status more closely. In cases in which the dura was violated, heavy bleeding occurred from the scalp edge, or the patient's underlying medical status is tenuous, an overnight stay in the intensive care unit is beneficial. However, for a routine cranioplasty, the authors obtain a postoperative computed tomographic scan and then place the patient in a non–intensive care setting. The subgaleal drain may be removed with the dressings on postoperative day 2.

COMPLICATIONS AFTER CRANIOPLASTY

Cranioplasty, although a routine neurosurgical procedure, can carry significant morbidity (**Table 2**), with rates of total major complications between 10.9% and 40.4% reported in the literature.[6,37] Choice of material used in cranioplasty does not seem to influence the rate of complications, although larger, prospective trials comparing various methods are needed.[38] It is also unclear whether or not timing of cranioplasty affects overall complication rates. Of note, the indication for cranioplasty may play a role in complication risk, with decompressive surgery for traumatic brain injury and stroke as predictors for perioperative morbidity.[39]

Autologous bone resorption may occur if the flap has become irreversibly devitalized or does

Table 2
Complication rates after cranioplasty

Complication	Incidence (%)
Overall complications	10.9–40.4[7–9,37,39]
Bone resorption	0.7–17.4[7,8,37,49]
Surgical site infection	5–12.8[7–9,37,39,49]
Seizure	3.4–14.8[9,39]
Hydrocephalus	1.4–5[7,9]
Postoperative hematoma	1.7–4.1[7,9,37,39]
Subdural hygroma formation	2.5[8]

From Piazza MA, Grady MS. Cranioplasty. In: Winn HR, editor. Youmans and Winn Neurological Surgery. 7th edition. Philadelphia: Elsevier; 2017:e154 with permission from Elsevier.

not come in contact with vascular native bone edge. This situation occurs when the soft tissue and scar tissue have not been adequately removed from the bone edge before replacement of the bone flap. Rates of bone resorption in the adult population vary from less than 1% to 17.4%.[8,37] Patients with comminuted skull fractures, fractures within the bone flap, or underlying brain contusion have higher rates of bone resorption; these factors may reflect the magnitude of force of injury and underlying microtrauma that devitalizes the bone flap.[40,41] Bone resorption seems to be more common in patients less than 18 years of age, with rates at or exceeding 50% reported in the literature.[40–42] Recent studies have shown reduced resorption rates when cranioplasty is performed early in this patient population.[43]

Surgical site infection is common after cranioplasty and rates as high as 21.7% have been reported in the literature.[6] Risk factors for surgical site infection include previous infection in the skull defect, communication between the operative site and cranial-facial sinuses, devascularized scalp, persistent subdural or subgaleal fluid collection, preoperative neurologic deficit, previous reoperation, and type of injury.[9,37,44] A recent study showed that implementing a perioperative cranioplasty protocol involving prolonged postoperative antibiotics and meticulous wound care was associated with lower rates of infection and cranioplasty revision.[45] In patients requiring multiple reoperations for bone flap infection, cranioplasty with antibiotic-impregnated methyl methacrylate flaps may be an effective salvage operation.[46]

Most patients undergoing cranioplasty already have epileptogenic brain tissue because of underlying injury that initially necessitates craniectomy, and unintended manipulation of brain during cranioplasty places these patients at even greater risk for seizures. Rates of postoperative seizure following cranioplasty between 3.4% and 14.8% have been reported.[9,39] The type of original injury, in particular intracerebral hemorrhage and trauma, as well as preoperative neurologic deficit, have been associated with greater rates of perioperative seizure and seem to reflect baseline epileptic predisposition.[39]

In most cases, cranioplasty improves CSF flow dynamics and restores normal intracranial pressure relationships within the skull.[47] However, in cases of traumatic brain injury or subarachnoid hemorrhage, the loss of brain parenchyma and obstruction of CSF pathways may not become apparent until after cranioplasty. Unilateral or bilateral subdural fluid collections may form if there has been intrinsic loss of brain parenchyma so that the brain does not fully reexpand to fill the skull. Attempts to decrease formation of these collections with subdural drains or central dural tacking sutures are not always successful. Similarly, the ventricles may increase in size after cranioplasty, either from brain atrophy or from manifesting true hydrocephalus. Typically, ventriculoperitoneal shunts are placed in a separate procedure to address these complications after the patient's neurologic status and clinical examination findings have stabilized after cranioplasty. Shunt placement at the time of cranioplasty is sometimes performed but carries a greater complication rate.[48]

SUMMARY

The need for cranioplasty will continue to increase as surgeons attempt resection of more aggressive tumors, acute emergency care continues to successfully resuscitate traumatic brain-injured patients, and the options for synthetic bone improve. However, unanswered questions remain regarding the optimal timing for cranioplasty and the physiologic and neurocognitive changes that accompany cranioplasty. In addition, despite the plethora of new materials used for cranioplasty, data comparing the various materials/methods with regard to clinical outcome, patient satisfaction, complication rates, and relative costs in the literature are lacking. Larger, prospective, multicenter studies are needed to answer these questions and will be instrumental in guiding neurosurgeons in clinical decision making.

REFERENCES

1. Grant FC, Norcross NC. Repair of cranial defects by cranioplasty. Ann Surg 1939;110(4):488–512.
2. Honeybul S, Janzen C, Kruger K, et al. The impact of cranioplasty on neurological function. Br J Neurosurg 2013;27(5):636–41.
3. Song J, Liu M, Mo X, et al. Beneficial impact of early cranioplasty in patients with decompressive craniectomy: evidence from transcranial Doppler ultrasonography. Acta Neurochir (Wien) 2014;156(1):193–8.
4. Kshettry VR, Hardy S, Weil RJ, et al. Immediate titanium cranioplasty after debridement and craniectomy for postcraniotomy surgical site infection. Neurosurgery 2012;70(1 Suppl Operative):8–14 [discussion: 14–5].
5. Baumeister S, Peek A, Friedman A, et al. Management of postneurosurgical bone flap loss caused by infection. Plast Reconstr Surg 2008;122(6):195e–208e.
6. Coulter IC, Pesic-Smith JD, Cato-Addison WB, et al. Routine but risky: a multi-centre analysis of the outcomes of cranioplasty in the northeast of England. Acta Neurochir (Wien) 2014;156(7):1361–8.
7. Piedra MP, Ragel BT, Dogan A, et al. Timing of cranioplasty after decompressive craniectomy for ischemic or hemorrhagic stroke. J Neurosurg 2013;118(1):109–14.
8. Wachter D, Reineke K, Behm T, et al. Cranioplasty after decompressive hemicraniectomy: underestimated surgery-associated complications? Clin Neurol Neurosurg 2013;115(8):1293–7.
9. Walcott BP, Kwon CS, Sheth SA, et al. Predictors of cranioplasty complications in stroke and trauma patients. J Neurosurg 2013;118(4):757–62.
10. Movassaghi K, Ver Halen J, Ganchi P, et al. Cranioplasty with subcutaneously preserved autologous bone grafts. Plast Reconstr Surg 2006;117(1):202–6.
11. Zingale A, Albanese V. Cryopreservation of autogeneous bone flap in cranial surgical practice: what is the future? A grade B and evidence level 4 meta-analytic study. J Neurosurg Sci 2003;47(3):137–9.
12. Prolo DJ, Burres KP, McLaughlin WT, et al. Autogenous skull cranioplasty: fresh and preserved (frozen), with consideration of the cellular response. Neurosurgery 1979;4(1):18–29.
13. Iwama T, Yamada J, Imai S, et al. The use of frozen autogenous bone flaps in delayed cranioplasty revisited. Neurosurgery 2003;52(3):591–6 [discussion: 595–6].
14. Grossman N, Shemesh-Jan HS, Merkin V, et al. Deep-freeze preservation of cranial bones for future cranioplasty: nine years of experience in Soroka University Medical Center. Cell Tissue Bank 2007;8(3):243–6.
15. Vignes JR, Jeelani N, Dautheribes M, et al. Cranioplasty for repair of a large bone defect in a growing skull fracture in children. J Craniomaxillofac Surg 2007;35(3):185–8.
16. Grant GA, Jolley M, Ellenbogen RG, et al. Failure of autologous bone-assisted cranioplasty following decompressive craniectomy in children and adolescents. J Neurosurg 2004;100(2 Suppl Pediatrics):163–8.
17. Jho DH, Neckrysh S, Hardman J, et al. Ethylene oxide gas sterilization: a simple technique for storing explanted skull bone. Technical note. J Neurosurg 2007;107(2):440–5.
18. Tamaki T, Eguchi T, Sakamoto M, et al. Use of diffusion-weighted magnetic resonance imaging in empyema after cranioplasty. Br J Neurosurg 2004;18(1):40–4.
19. Chiang HY, Steelman VM, Pottinger JM, et al. Clinical significance of positive cranial bone flap cultures and associated risk of surgical site infection after craniotomies or craniectomies. J Neurosurg 2011;114(6):1746–54.
20. Lake PA, Morin MA, Pitts FW. Radiolucent prosthesis of mesh-reinforced acrylic. Technical note. J Neurosurg 1970;32(5):597–602.

21. Blum KS, Schneider SJ, Rosenthal AD. Methyl methacrylate cranioplasty in children: long-term results. Pediatr Neurosurg 1997;26(1):33–5.

22. Marchac D, Greensmith A. Long-term experience with methylmethacrylate cranioplasty in craniofacial surgery. J Plast Reconstr Aesthet Surg 2008;61(7):744–52 [discussion: 753].

23. Nisbet M, Briggs S, Ellis-Pegler R, et al. *Propionibacterium acnes*: an under-appreciated cause of post-neurosurgical infection. J Antimicrob Chemother 2007;60(5):1097–103.

24. Edwards SA, Gardiner J. Hypersensitivity to benzoyl peroxide in a cemented total knee arthroplasty: cement allergy. J Arthroplasty 2007;22(8):1226–8.

25. Newens AF, Volz RG. Severe hypotension during prosthetic hip surgery with acrylic bone cement. Anesthesiology 1972;36(3):298–300.

26. Kubo S, Takimoto H, Kato A, et al. Endoscopic cranioplasty with calcium phosphate cement for pterional bone defect after frontotemporal craniotomy: technical note. Neurosurgery 2002;51(4):1094–6 [discussion: 1096].

27. Miyake H, Ohta T, Tanaka H. A new technique for cranioplasty with L-shaped titanium plates and combination ceramic implants composed of hydroxyapatite and tricalcium phosphate (Ceratite). Neurosurgery 2000;46(2):414–8.

28. Miller L, Guerra AB, Bidros RS, et al. A comparison of resistance to fracture among four commercially available forms of hydroxyapatite cement. Ann Plast Surg 2005;55(1):87–92 [discussion: 93].

29. Li G, Wen L, Zhan RY, et al. Cranioplasty for patients developing large cranial defects combined with post-traumatic hydrocephalus after head trauma. Brain Inj 2008;22(4):333–7.

30. Marbacher S, Andres RH, Fathi AR, et al. Primary reconstruction of open depressed skull fractures with titanium mesh. J Craniofac Surg 2008;19(2):490–5.

31. Chim H, Schantz JT. New frontiers in calvarial reconstruction: integrating computer-assisted design and tissue engineering in cranioplasty. Plast Reconstr Surg 2005;116(6):1726–41.

32. Winder J, Cooke RS, Gray J, et al. Medical rapid prototyping and 3D CT in the manufacture of custom made cranial titanium plates. J Med Eng Technol 1999;23(1):26–8.

33. Eufinger H, Wehmoller M. Individual prefabricated titanium implants in reconstructive craniofacial surgery: clinical and technical aspects of the first 22 cases. Plast Reconstr Surg 1998;102(2):300–8.

34. Liu JK, Gottfried ON, Cole CD, et al. Porous polyethylene implant for cranioplasty and skull base reconstruction. Neurosurg Focus 2004;16(3):ECP1.

35. Pietrzak WS, Eppley BL. Antibiotic elution from hydroxyapatite cement cranioplasty materials. J Craniofac Surg 2005;16(2):228–33.

36. Itokawa H, Hiraide T, Moriya M, et al. A 12 month in vivo study on the response of bone to a hydroxyapatite-polymethylmethacrylate cranioplasty composite. Biomaterials 2007;28(33):4922–7.

37. Klinger D, Madden C, Beshay J, et al. Autologous and acrylic cranioplasty: a review of 10 years and 258 cases. World Neurosurg 2014;82:e525–30.

38. Yadla S, Campbell PG, Chitale R, et al. Effect of early surgery, material, and method of flap preservation on cranioplasty infections: a systematic review. Neurosurgery 2011;68(4):1124–9 [discussion: 1130].

39. Lee L, Ker J, Quah BL, et al. A retrospective analysis and review of an institution's experience with the complications of cranioplasty. Br J Neurosurg 2013;27(5):629–35.

40. Schuss P, Vatter H, Oszvald A, et al. Bone flap resorption: risk factors for the development of a long-term complication following cranioplasty after decompressive craniectomy. J Neurotrauma 2013;30(2):91–5.

41. Bowers CA, Riva-Cambrin J, Hertzler DA 2nd, et al. Risk factors and rates of bone flap resorption in pediatric patients after decompressive craniectomy for traumatic brain injury. J Neurosurg Pediatr 2013;11(5):526–32.

42. Martin KD, Franz B, Kirsch M, et al. Autologous bone flap cranioplasty following decompressive craniectomy is combined with a high complication rate in pediatric traumatic brain injury patients. Acta Neurochir (Wien) 2014;156(4):813–24.

43. Piedra MP, Thompson EM, Selden NR, et al. Optimal timing of autologous cranioplasty after decompressive craniectomy in children. J Neurosurg Pediatr 2012;10(4):268–72.

44. Rengachary S, Benzel E. Calvarial and dural reconstruction. Park Ridge (IL): AANS; 1998.

45. Le C, Guppy KH, Axelrod YV, et al. Lower complication rates for cranioplasty with peri-operative bundle. Clin Neurol Neurosurg 2014;120:41–4.

46. Hsu VM, Tahiri Y, Wilson AJ, et al. A preliminary report on the use of antibiotic-impregnated methyl methacrylate in salvage cranioplasty. J Craniofac Surg 2014;25(2):393–6.

47. Waziri A, Fusco D, Mayer SA, et al. Postoperative hydrocephalus in patients undergoing decompressive hemicraniectomy for ischemic or hemorrhagic stroke. Neurosurgery 2007;61(3):489–93 [discussion: 493–4].

48. Heo J, Park SQ, Cho SJ, et al. Evaluation of simultaneous cranioplasty and ventriculoperitoneal shunt procedures. J Neurosurg 2014;121:313–8.

49. Sundseth J, Sundseth A, Berg-Johnsen J, et al. Cranioplasty with autologous cryopreserved bone after decompressive craniectomy. Complications and risk factors for developing surgical site infection. Acta Neurochir (Wien) 2014;156(4):805–11 [discussion: 811].

Neurocritical Care of Acute Subdural Hemorrhage

Fawaz Al-Mufti, MD[a], Stephan A. Mayer, MD[b],*

KEYWORDS

- Acute subdural hematoma • Acute subdural hemorrhage • Traumatic brain injury
- Advanced Trauma Life Support protocol

KEY POINTS

- Although urgent surgical hematoma evacuation is necessary for most patients with SDH, well-orchestrated, evidenced-based, multidisciplinary, postoperative critical care is essential to achieve the best possible outcome.
- Acute SDH complicates approximately 11% of mild to moderate traumatic brain injuries (TBIs) that require hospitalization, and approximately 20% of severe TBIs.
- In most cases, acute SDH is related to a clear traumatic event, but in some cases, acute SDH can occur spontaneously.
- Management of SDH in the setting of TBI typically conforms to the Advanced Trauma Life Support (ATLS) protocol with airway taking priority, and management breathing and circulation occurring in parallel rather than in sequence.

INTRODUCTION

Acute subdural hematoma (SDH) develops between the dura and arachnoid membranes, usually due to tearing of the bridging veins that extend from the surface of the brain to the dural sinuses. Most cases of SDH result from low-pressure venous bleeding that eventually arrests due to rising intracranial pressure (ICP) and clot tamponade, but it is estimated that up to 20% to 30% of cases can result from arterial rupture.[1–3] Linear translation of acceleration across the diameter of the skull in the lateral direction can produce stretch or torque injury to veins or arteries, resulting in SDH.[4]

Acute SDH complicates approximately 11% of mild to moderate traumatic brain injuries (TBIs) that require hospitalization, and approximately 20% of severe TBIs.[5–8] In most cases, acute

SDH is related to a clear traumatic event, but in some cases acute SDH can occur spontaneously. Important causes of spontaneous SDH include use of anticoagulants or antiplatelet agents, and rupture of an intracranial aneurysm that is adherent to the arachnoid membrane, with consequent arterial bleeding into the subdural space (with or without associated subarachnoid hemorrhage).[9–11] Less commonly, SDH also can result from bleeding due to arteriovenous malformations, vascular meningiomas, dural metastases, and spontaneous intracranial hypotension.[12–14] Identification of a treatable cause of nontraumatic SDH is crucial, because reversal of anticoagulation may be all that is necessary in some patients, whereas others may require treatment of a cerebral aneurysm.

After traumatic acute SDH, coma is present at the onset of injury in 25% to 50% of cases,

[a] Endovascular Surgical Neuroradiology Program, Rutgers University-New Jersey Medical School, Newark, NJ, USA; [b] Department of Neurology, Henry Ford Health System, 2799 W Grand Boulevard, Detroit, MI 48202, USA
* Corresponding author.
E-mail address: stephanamayer@gmail.com

Neurosurg Clin N Am 28 (2017) 267–278
http://dx.doi.org/10.1016/j.nec.2016.11.009

whereas another 12% to 38% experience progressive neurologic decline to coma over the next several hours.[15,16] Coma is primarily the result of brain shifting and distortion, followed by elevated ICP and low cerebral perfusion pressure (CPP).[17] Large acute SDH leads to compression and ischemia of the underlying brain within 4 to 6 hours in the absence of emergency evacuation.[18] Posterior fossa SDH is especially treacherous because it can precipitate upward or downward herniation extremely rapidly.[19]

EMERGENCY RESUSCITATION
Airway, Breathing, Circulation

The objectives in the emergency department are to undertake a rapid and systematic clinical assessment, and to institute immediate lifesaving treatment. Management of SDH in the setting of TBI typically conforms to the Advanced Trauma Life Support (ATLS) protocol, with airway taking priority, and management breathing and circulation occurring in parallel rather than in sequence.[20] As is the case with all forms of severe trauma, maintenance of oxygenation (Pao_2 >60 mm Hg) and blood pressure (BP) at a mean arterial pressure (MAP) of 65 mm Hg or higher is the immediate priority.[21]

Deciding on the optimal timing to secure the airway can be challenging. Intubation and ventilation may allow for expedited imaging, as well as safer interventions in the unconscious or agitated patient.[22] Intubations in the setting of TBI and elevated ICP are more challenging, with higher rates of failure and complications.[23] As a general rule, rapid sequence intubation (RSI) after an initial period of preoxygenation is the preferred strategy.[24–26] RSI is the concomitant administration of a sedative and a neuromuscular blocking agent to render a patient rapidly unconscious and flaccid so as to facilitate emergent endotracheal intubation and to minimize the risk of aspiration. Multiple studies confirm the high first-pass success rate of RSI, which in experienced hands can exceed 90%.[25,26]

Induction agents provide amnesia and blunt sympathetic responses, and can improve intubating conditions. Pretreatment with intravenous (IV) lidocaine 1.5 mg/kg 3 minutes before intubation may minimize any increase in ICP that can be associated with airway manipulation. Ketamine 1.5 mg/kg IV or etomidate 0.3 mg/kg are suitable induction agents because they tend to maintain MAP and do not increase ICP. Ketamine is a dissociative anesthetic agent that provides sedation and analgesia. Ketamine preserves respiratory drive and has both a quick onset of action and analgesic properties.[27] Ketamine can cause sympathetic stimulation, and although it is known to maintain BP, there is concern that it may cause ICP elevation in TBI.[28,29] Etomidate is a sedative-hypnotic agent that is frequently used for RSI that has putative neuroprotective properties.[30] It provides no analgesic effect, so it often is given with fentanyl 1.5 μg/kg, administered during the pretreatment phase of RSI. For paralysis, a short-acting paralytic, such as succinylcholine 1.5 mg/kg IV, is ideal, because it wears off quickly and restores the neurologic examination within 10 to 15 minutes (use with caution in the setting of crush injury or hyperkalemia).

Longer-acting nondepolarizing alternatives include rocuronium (0.6–1.2 mg/kg) or cisatracurium (0.15 mg/kg).

Imaging

Neuroimaging in the form of a noncontrast computed tomography (CT) is integral to the diagnosis of acute SDH due to it widespread availability and speed. The sensitivity now approaches 100% with newer generation scanners.[31] Brain MRI is more sensitive than head CT for the detection of extremely thin SDH, and tentorial and interhemispheric SDH.[31] Acute SDH can be classified by (1) the age of the imaged blood (eg, acute, acute-on-subacute, or acute-on-chronic), and (2) by the maximal thickness of the subdural collection in centimeters (**Fig. 1**). Additional parameters to assess are the extent of midline shift, the presence of effacement of the basal cisterns, and the extent of trapping of the contralateral ventricle. Because SDH can result from a ruptured cerebral aneurysm, noninvasive or digital subtraction angiography should be performed in suspicious cases of nontraumatic acute SDH.

Reversal of Anticoagulation

Reversal of all forms of anticoagulation is a medical emergency in patients with acute SDH. Coagulation panels are typically obtained on arrival; whether or not the patient is on some form of anticoagulation or antiplatelet therapy should be discerned through the history. The Neurocritical Care Society has published the most up-to-date guidelines for the emergency reversal of anticoagulation.[32] Patients on oral anticoagulation therapy are estimated to have a 4- to 15-fold increased risk for SDH, leading to higher likelihood of hematoma expansion, an increased risk of death, and a worse functional outcome unless anticoagulation is quickly reversed.[33,34] Patients on vitamin K antagonists, such as warfarin, are optimally reversed with vitamin K 10 mg

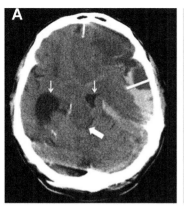 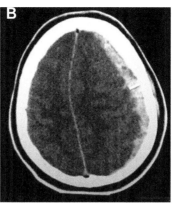

Fig. 1. Two images of acute SDH. (*A*) A massive acute-on-chronic SDH with effacement of the quadrigeminal cistern (*thick arrow*) and trapping of both temporal horns of the lateral ventricles (*thin arrows*). The white bar shows the maximal lateral diameter (2.5 cm) of the collection (the diameter is not measured in the frontal region because at this level the plane of the collection is parallel to the plane of the image). (*B*) A 1-cm acute SDH with lateral bowing of the falx tentorium from left to right.

intravenous push, followed by a 4-factor prothrombin complex concentrate (PCC) (Kentraor BeriplexV; CSL Behring, Inc, King of Prussia, PA) at a dose of 25 U/kg for an international normalized ratio (INR) of 2.0 to 4.0, 35 U/kg for an INR of 4.0 to 6.0, and 50 U/kg for an INR greater than 6.0. Recombinant factor VIIa (rFVIIa, NovoSeven; Novo Nordisk, Copenhagen, Denmark) was studied in TBI a phase II dose-escalation clinical trial and demonstrated a nonsignificant trend toward limiting hematoma contusion and hematoma expansion but no mortality benefit.[35] rFVIIa also has been reported to be useful for emergency reversal of warfarin anticoagulation in patients with acute SDH.[36] Given the associated risk of thromboembolic complications, however, routine use of rFVIIa cannot be recommended.[32]

SDH associated with the newer direct oral anticoagulants (DOACs), such as the direct thrombin inhibitor dabigatran and the Factor Xa inhibitors, such as apixaban, edoxaban, and rivaroxaban, can lead to catastrophic bleeding, but until recently have had no antidote for emergency reversal.[37] That has now changed with the arrival of idarucizumab (Praxbind; Boehringer Ingelheim, Ingelheim am Rhein, Germany) for dabigatran, which is currently approved by the Food and Drug Administration (FDA), and andexanet alfa (IndexXa; Portola Pharmaceuticals, San Francisco, CA) for the direct Factor Xa inhibitors, which is pending FDA approval.[32]

Patients with acute subdural hematoma on antiplatelet agents should be managed initially by discontinuing antiplatelet therapy.[38] Although platelet transfusion has long been considered a standard of care in the absence of evidence, the recently published PATCH trial compared platelet transfusion versus standard care after acute spontaneous intracerebral hemorrhage associated with antiplatelet therapy.[39] This study demonstrated an

increased risk of death or dependence at 3 months with platelet transfusion, and a *higher* rate of adverse events, with platelet transfusion. The Neurocritical Care Society recommends against platelet transfusion regardless of the type of platelet inhibitor, platelet function testing, hemorrhage volume, or neurologic examination.[32] However, in patients who will undergo a neurosurgical procedure, it is reasonable to correct thrombocytopenia to maintain a level greater than 75,000.[40] Additionally a single dose of desmopressin (DDAVP) in patients with antiplatelet-associated intracranial hemorrhage has been recommended (0.4 μg/kg IV), despite the lack of level 1 evidence in patients with intracranial hemorrhage supporting its use.[41–43]

Severe coagulopathy has been demonstrated in approximately 30% of patients who sustain severe TBI. This is believed to occur due to the systemic release of tissue factor and brain phospholipids into the circulation, leading to disseminated intravascular coagulation and a consumptive coagulopathy.[44,45] The process is exacerbated by acidosis, hypothermia, and excessive crystalloid administration. Correction of these metabolic abnormalities, along with replacement of fibrinogen and coagulation factors with cryoprecipitate and plasma or a PCC, is the only known treatment.

CRITICAL CARE MANAGEMENT
Intracranial Pressure Monitoring and Treatment

Elevated ICP is associated with increased mortality and worsened outcome after TBI.[16,17] *Clinical studies indicate that ICP is most highly elevated before surgical SDH evacuation, making empiric treatment of intracranial hypertension during the acute period crucial. In one study of 5 patients* who were monitored before surgical hematoma evacuation, ICP ranged from 40 to 85 mm Hg and CPP ranged from 5 to 56 mm Hg before craniotomy.[46] Craniotomy resulted in dramatic ICP reductions, and immediate improvement of cerebral blood flow (CBF) and jugular venous oxygen saturation, indicative of improved cerebral perfusion.

Clinical signs, such as decline in level of consciousness, unilaterally dilated or poorly responsive pupils, or extensor posturing, are signs that a patient is actively undergoing brainstem herniation and requires emergent management. Several techniques have been developed to abort signs and symptoms of herniation. The head of the bed should be elevated 30° to improve venous drainage, and care should be taken to ensure that there is no apparatus near or around the neck (such as a constrictive C-spine collar) blocking venous drainage.[16] Hyperventilation lowers ICP by inducing vasoconstriction, although care should be taken to avoid excessive respiratory alkalosis, which may exacerbate secondary ischemia.[47–49] In one randomized study, patients with TBI hyperventilated to a $Paco_2$ of 25 mm Hg for 5 days had a worse clinical outcome than nonhyperventilated controls.[50] Hyperventilation may be used to target a $Paco_2$ of 30 mm Hg, and is best used for brief periods due to a wearing off effect that can occur.[16] In a study of 75 patients with acute SDH studied with Xenon CBF, almost all had demonstrated reactive hyperemia postoperatively, which was related to ICP elevation and responsive to controlled hyperventilation.[51]

Bolus osmolar therapy can be initiated with mannitol 1.0 to 1.5 g/kg and/or 30 to 120 mL of 23.4% hypertonic saline. In a study of 178 patients with acute SDH comparing low-dose and high-dose mannitol, the higher dose (1.4 g/kg) was associated with more frequent reversal of pupillary abnormalities, and lower ICP and better clinical outcome postoperatively.[52] The osmotic gradient created by these agents favors efflux of interstitial and intracellular fluid across capillaries and into the circulation, thus reducing brain tissue water content and volume. There is no proven efficacy of targeting a particular sodium level (eg, sodium >155 mEq/L), and no evidence that hyperosmolar therapy loses its efficacy once a given serum osmolality level has been reached (eg, osmolality >320 mOsm/L).[16] Highly elevated sodium levels (>165 mEq/L) have been associated with poor outcome, but this most likely reflects the severity of the primary injury, more than any particular harm caused by the hypernatremia itself. Because hypertonic saline increases intravascular volume and BP, it should be used in favor of mannitol in patients who are dehydrated, hypovolemic, or hypotensive. Conversely, hypertonic saline should be avoided in favor of mannitol in patients who are fluid overloaded or who have congestive heart failure.[16]

In addition to its neuroprotective effects, hypothermia has been shown to decrease metabolic demand and ICP through reductions in cerebral blood volume and edema. A recent randomized controlled trial (EuroTherm 32–34) examining the effects of hypothermia (32–34°C) at the first sign of intracranial hypertension after TBI showed efficacy with regard to reduction of ICP and the need for barbiturate coma and decompressive hemicraniectomy, but not with regard to clinical outcome: in fact, outcomes were worse in patients who underwent systemic cooling.[53] The reason for the worsening of outcome in the intervention arm was not apparent, however, because there was no marked increase in adverse events, such as infection or arrhythmia in the hypothermia group. An important criticism of this trial is that the intervention arm did not reflect standard practice, because hypothermia is typically reserved for cases of ICP refractory to cerebrospinal fluid drainage, sedation, CPP optimization, hyperventilation, and repeated doses of bolus osmotherapy. Based on these data, hypothermia cannot be recommended as a form of salvage therapy for elevated ICP after TBI.

Seizure Prophylaxis

Up to 24% of patients with traumatic SDH develop seizures either on presentation or postoperatively.[54] Prophylactic antiepileptic drugs (AEDs) reduce the frequency of early seizures, which can increase metabolic demand and increase ICP.[55,56] In the most widely cited trial, prophylactic phenytoin after TBI reduced the frequency of early seizures from 14% to 4%.[55] An observational study found an even greater effect, with 2% of patients with TBI who received prophylactic anticonvulsant medications developing seizures, compared with 32% who did not.[57]

In practice, phenytoin/fosphenytoin is frequently used because it can be loaded intravenously and does not cause significant sedation. Levetiracetam has recently become a popular alternative due to its more favorable adverse effect profile.[58] In a randomized controlled trial and an observational study, there was no difference between phenytoin or levetiracetam in terms of reducing the rates of early seizures and adverse drug reactions.[59,60]

The use of prophylactic AEDs does not reduce the risk of late seizures or posttraumatic epilepsy.[55] Large-scale trials examining the optimal duration of seizure prophylaxis are lacking. AEDs are generally continued throughout the hospital stay, and in the absence of documented seizures, can be safely stopped before discharge, to avoid the deleterious effects that un-needed AEDs can have on neural recovery during rehabilitation.

Glucocorticoids

There is no limited evidence supporting the routine use of glucocorticoids in TBI. In fact, the use of glucocorticoid therapy was found to be harmful in large, prospective, randomized multicenter trials of patients with moderate to severe TBI.[61]

Ventilatory Support

Hypercapnia and hypoxia can be detrimental in patients with neurologic emergencies; hence, early securement of the airway and optimal ventilation are crucial.[62,63] Furthermore, mechanical ventilation allows for safer use of sedation. Postintubation sedation with propofol, midazolam, or dexmedetomidine has been found to help prevent neuroexcitation (ie, autonomic storming) and ventilator dyssynchrony. Lung protective ventilation strategies that use low tidal volume ventilation (4–8 mL/kg) and often permissive hypercapnia, should be used only when ICP is monitored to ensure that hypercapnia is not contributing to intracranial hypertension.[64,65] Iatrogenic hyperventilation therapy ($Paco_2$ $\leq$35 mm Hg) after TBI may compromise CPP at a time when CBF may already be critically educed.[64] A small study examining the effects of varying levels of positive end-expiratory pressure (PEEP) in coma patients failed to show a uniform effect of higher levels of PEEP (10–15 cm H_2O) on ICP or CPP.[66] In another study, high PEEP (10–15 cm H_2O) levels increased brain tissue oxygen tension (PbtO2) and oxygen saturation, without increase in ICP or decrease in CPP.[67]

Little is known about the effect of prolonged mechanical ventilation in patients with SDH. One study reported that prolonged mechanical ventilation was associated with pulmonary complications, increased length of stay, and unfavorable discharge destination in patients.[68] These complications were primarily seen in patients with history of alcohol abuse, low admission Glasgow Coma Score (GCS), and patients who required surgical evacuation.

Blood Pressure and Cerebral Perfusion Pressure Management

Normal cerebral autoregulation maintains an optimal CBF across a wide range of BP.[69–72] It is estimated that 30% of patients with SDH in the setting of severe TBI have impaired cerebral autoregulation.[72] Accordingly, avoidance of wide fluctuations in BP has been thought to be beneficial, because extremes of CPP can lead to increases in ICP (Fig. 2) and worse clinical outcomes.[73,74] Before evacuation, given the tendency of cerebral infarction to develop in the underlying brain, it seems wisest to avoid any kind of BP reduction. After hematoma evacuation, given the risk of postoperative bleeding into friable tissues and the empty subdural space, it has been suggested that lowering the systolic BPs to approximately 140 mm Hg may be beneficial, as is the case with hypertensive intracerebral hemorrhage (ICH), but this remains speculative.[75]

In patients with ICP monitoring, BP management should be based on CPP targets. As a

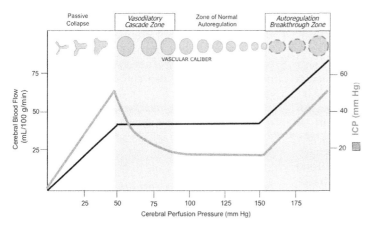

Fig. 2. Cerebral autoregulation curve and relationship between CPP and ICP in states of abnormal intracranial compliance. Under normal circumstances, CBF is held constant across a wide range of CPP (50–150 mm Hg), and changes in vessel caliber have no effect on ICP. In disease states with reduced intracranial compliance, ICP can become elevated when CPP is low due to autoregulatory vasodilation and increased cerebral blood volume (vasodilatory cascade physiology) or when CPP is too high due to passive increases in CBV due to increased hydrostatic pressure and hyperemia (autoregulation breakthrough physiology). For this reason, it is advisable to avoid extremes of BP in patients with TBI and acute SDH.

general rule, CPP should be maintained above 60 mm Hg in adults and in the range of 40 to 65 mm Hg in children.[76–78] Efforts to optimize CPP should first always start with ICP reduction, if it is elevated.[79] From the cardiac perspective, although acute SDH may be associated with electrocardiogram (ECG) abnormalities, myocardial injury and stunning are infrequent.[80]

Analgosedation

Sedation and analgesia are integral to the management of acute SDH to minimize ventilator dyssynchrony and blunt sympathetic responses. Although this is largely beneficial, analgosedation can produce hypotension and potentially cerebral hypoperfusion. As a general rule, sedation always should conform to 3 basic principles.[81] First, pain always should be treated first. Second, the level of sedation should be targeted to clinical response using scales such as the Richmond Sedation Agitation Scale or the Riker Sedation Agitation Scale. Third, sedation should be interrupted on a regular (at least daily) basis to assess neurologic status and to determine the minimum amount of sedation required moving forward. The only exception to the third rule is when dangerous agitation, refractory ICP, or severe hypoxia might result from a "wake-up" test.

Fentanyl and remifentanil are powerful opioid agents that are useful continuous infusion agents for establishing an adequate level of analgesia.[81] Fentanyl is typically given at 25 to 200 µg/h. Remifentanil has an even faster onset and offset of sedation, making it ideal for neurologic checks, and is given in the range of 0.5 to 2.0 µg/kg per minute. Disadvantages of these opioid agents include hypotension, ileus, and opioid withdrawal after prolonged infusions.

Propofol is an attractive agent to use in acute SDH because of its rapid onset and offset, which makes intermittent neurologic evaluations easier. It can easily be added to a baseline fentanyl infusion to attain a given sedation goal. Propofol also suppresses cerebral metabolism and may lower ICP while also conferring some neuroprotective effects.[82] Propofol is started at a rate of 5 µg/kg per minute (or 0.3 mg/kg per hour) and titrated by increments of increase by 5 to 10 µg/kg per minute (or 0.3–0.6 mg/kg per hour) until desired sedation level is achieved. Significant concerns when using propofol include respiratory suppression, hypotension, infections with prolonged infusions, and propofol infusion syndrome (PRIS).[83] PRIS is a rare but potentially lethal complication seen more frequently with sepsis, serious cerebral injury, and the administration of high doses of propofol

(usually doses >83 µg/kg per minute or >5 mg/kg per hour for >48 hours). It is associated with a high mortality rate (up to 33%) and is clinically characterized by circulatory collapse, metabolic acidosis, rhabdomyolysis or myoglobinuria with renal failure, dysrhythmias, and hyperkalemia. As a result, it is suggested that when used in TBI, the infusion rate of propofol not exceed 4 mg/kg per hour and that patients be monitored for ECG changes, lactic acidosis, and elevations in creatinine kinase and myoglobin. Because propofol is delivered in a lipid vehicle, some advocate adjusting dietary calories so as to avoid overfeeding.

Midazolam also is routinely used for inducing sedation in patients with TBI; it is a potent and short-acting benzodiazepine with sedative and amnestic, but not analgesic, effects. It is particularly useful as an add-on to fentanyl in patients with seizures or alcohol withdrawal. The advantages of midazolam are its rapid onset, easy titration, water solubility, and circumvention of the metabolic acidosis associated with the propylene glycol vehicle of other benzodiazepines, such as lorazepam.[84,85] The major disadvantage of midazolam is the development of tachyphylaxis with prolonged infusions, and the potential for benzodiazepines to cause delirium.[84] One meta-analysis of 4 studies showed that there are no important differences between propofol and midazolam when administered to provide sedation for patients with severe TBI.[85] Dexmedetomidine also may be used as a primary agent or as an adjunct to opioids for sedation.[86] It is a selective centrally acting alpha-2-agonist with anxiolytic, sedative, and some analgesic effects and no deleterious effects on respiratory drive. It is particularly effective for its sympatholytic effects in patients with TBI with autonomic storming. An initial loading dose is typically not required and a typical maintenance dose is 0.2 to 0.7 µg/kg per hour, with dosage increases no more frequently than every 30 minutes. Doses greater than 1.5 µg/kg per hour do not appear to add to the clinical efficacy of dexmedetomidine.[87,88] Potential adverse effects of dexmedetomidine include bradycardia, hypotension, and nausea.[87]

A meta-analysis of randomized controlled trials found no conclusive mortality benefit associated with the use of any particular analgosedative agent in patients with TBI.[89]

Follow-up Imaging and Advanced Neuromonitoring

After hematoma evacuation, follow-up serial imaging is critical to ensure that recurrent hematoma formation is addressed promptly. Immediate postoperative imaging is important to establish a baseline, and subsequent imaging may be indicated with any deterioration in neurologic examination. Follow-up imaging within 1 to 2 weeks is also commonly pursued in otherwise asymptomatic patients to monitor for signs of progression or recurrence.

After surgical evacuation, management of patients with severe SDH who are comatose focuses on detection and management of neurologic complications. Multimodality neurologic monitoring has emerged as a promising tool in detecting subclinical deleterious physiologic changes by tracking oxygen delivery, CBF, and metabolism with the goal of improving the detection and management of secondary brain injury. Jugular venous oximetry (SjvO2) allows measurement of oxygen saturation in the venous blood exiting the brain.[90] SjvO2 provides information on the global cerebral utilization of oxygen. Normal values range from 60% to 90%; an SjvO2 less than 50% represents cerebral ischemia and is associated with low CPP and worsened outcome, whereas SjvO2 values greater than 90% are indicative of hyperemia.[91,92]

PbtO2 can be measured using intraparenchymal probes placed in white matter, at a depth of approximately 3 cm.[93] Normal thresholds of PbtO2 range from 30 to 40 mm Hg, with values lower than 15 mm Hg being associated with poor outcome.[94] One case series used oxygen supplementation to maintain PbtO2 higher than 25 mm Hg and found better outcomes compared with historical controls.[95]

Cerebral microdialysis measures extracellular glucose, lactate, pyruvate, and glutamate.[96] Lactate-to-pyruvate ratios are normally 40; ratios less than 20 indicate metabolic distress and enhanced anaerobic metabolism.[97,98]

Invasive multimodality monitoring can improve real-time situational awareness of secondary brain injury, and allows intensivists to individualize management, including BP, temperature, and serum glucose levels.

Deep Vein Thrombosis Prophylaxis

Deep vein thrombosis (DVT) prophylaxis with low molecular weight heparin or unfractionated heparin should be initiated shortly after admission for SDH, as DVT and pulmonary embolism account for significant morbidity and mortality in bed-bound patients with stroke. Low molecular weight heparin is more effective than unfractionated heparin in preventing DVT. Although there are no randomized controlled trials analyzing the optimal time to start DVT prophylaxis in patients with hemorrhage, it is reasonable to start most patients at 24 to 48 hours

after the initial event when an non-contrast CT scan head shows stability of the bleed.[99,100]

Temperature Management

Extrapolating from the TBI and general critical care literature, normothermia should be the goal temperature for patients with acute SDH. Hyperthermia in patients with neurologic emergencies has been associated with increase in mortality in the first 24 hours after hospitalization, presumably by aggravating secondary brain injury.[10] The evaluation of fever should include an infectious workup to rule out pulmonary and urinary tract infections as well as bacteremia. Central fever, defined as noninfectious temperature elevation due to disturbances in the central mechanisms of thermoregulation, should remain a diagnosis of exclusion. Once the workup and treatment of the underlying cause of fevers has been initiated, core body temperature should be reduced, either with direct cooling or pharmacologic means. Acetaminophen should be used first, followed by ibuprofen. Refractory fevers may require cooling devices for adequate control, which may necessitate active control of shiverin.[101]

Blood Glucose Control

Avoiding severe hyperglycemia is reasonable in patients with SDH, as it is among all critically ill patients, and in general this can be achieved by using insulin sliding scales. It is reasonable to maintain glucose levels of 120 to 180 mg/dL in patients in the ICU.[102] Microdialysis monitoring of patients with severe TBI has shown that critical brain tissue hypoglycemia can occur with tight glycemic control, however.[103] In these patients, higher serum glucose targets, titrated to brain extracellular glucose levels, may be desirable.

Fluids and Nutrition

Several factors should be considered with regard to fluid composition and the optimal volume infused. Existing guidelines suggest targeting euvolemia using isotonic fluids such as 0.9% (normal) saline or a balanced solution such as Plasmalyte. Hypotonic fluids, such as half-normal saline or D5W, may cause water shifts across the blood–brain barrier (BBB), potentially exacerbating cerebral edema and ICP.[104–106] Aggressive fluid administration aimed at hypervolemia is considered harmful due to the increased risk of lung injury and acute respiratory distress syndrome (ARDS), and should be avoided.[107]

Adequate nutritional support should be instituted as soon as possible (eg, usually after 24–48 hours) because early enteral feeding after TBI has been shown to improve outcome compared with delayed feeding. A hypermetabolic, catabolic response may develop in patients with traumatic SDH leading to caloric requirements that are 50% to 100% higher than normal.[108] Estimates of daily caloric requirements are important, because both underfeeding and overfeeding are associated with complications.[109]

Stress Ulcer Prophylaxis

Gastrointestinal (GI) hemorrhage is a serious complication and potential cause of mortality in critically ill neurologic patients. Although the frequency of stress ulcer–related GI bleeding is relatively low, patients at risk for GI bleeds include those on a mechanical ventilator, patients who are comatose, and patients with coagulopathy or a previous history of GI bleeding.[110] In one study of 51 patients with intracranial hemorrhage that included patients with SDH, the size of the hematoma, development of septicemia, and lower GCS scores were found to be predictors of GI hemorrhages.[111] Although the optimal agent for acid suppression is unknown, both H2 receptor blockers and proton pump inhibitors are considered agents of choice. For critically ill patients who are able to receive enteral medications, oral proton pump inhibitors are preferred over histamine-2 receptor antagonists, sucralfate, or antacids. In cases in which enteral medications are contraindicated, an IV histamine-2 receptor antagonist or IV proton pump inhibitor can be administered.[112,113]

SUMMARY

Although urgent surgical hematoma evacuation is necessary for most patients with SDH, well-orchestrated, evidenced-based, multidisciplinary, postoperative critical care is essential to achieve the best possible outcome.

REFERENCES

1. Gennarelli TA, Thlbault LE. Biomechanics of acute subdural hematoma. J Trauma 1982;22:680–6.
2. Haselsberger K, Pucher R, Auer LM. Prognosis after acute subdural or epidural haemorrhage. Acta Neurochir 1988;90:111–6.
3. Maxeiner H, Wolff M. Pure subdural hematomas: a postmortem analysis of their form and bleeding points. Neurosurgery 2002;50:503–8 [discussion: 508–9].
4. Besenski N. Traumatic injuries: imaging of head injuries. Eur Radiol 2002;12:1237–52.
5. Bullock MR, Chesnut R, Ghajar J, et al. Surgical management of acute subdural hematomas. Neurosurgery 2006;58:S16–24 [discussion: Si–iv].
6. Massaro F, Lanotte M, Faccani G, et al. One hundred and twenty-seven cases of acute subdural haematoma operated on. Correlation between CT scan findings and outcome. Acta Neurochir 1996;138:185–91.
7. Servadei F, Nasi MT, Giuliani G, et al. CT prognostic factors in acute subdural haematomas: the value of the 'worst' CT scan. Br J Neurosurg 2000;14:110–6.
8. Servadei F, Nasi MT, Cremonini AM, et al. Importance of a reliable admission Glasgow coma scale score for determining the need for evacuation of posttraumatic subdural hematomas: a prospective study of 65 patients. J Trauma 1998;44:868–73.
9. Inamasu J, Saito R, Nakamura Y, et al. Acute subdural hematoma caused by ruptured cerebral aneurysms: diagnostic and therapeutic pitfalls. Resuscitation 2002;52:71–6.
10. Rengachary SS, Szymanski DC. Subdural hematomas of arterial origin. Neurosurgery 1981;8:166–72.
11. Hylek EM, Singer DE. Risk factors for intracranial hemorrhage in outpatients taking warfarin. Ann Intern Med 1994;120:897–902.
12. Okuno S, Touho H, Ohnishi H, et al. Falx meningioma presenting as acute subdural hematoma: case report. Surg Neurol 1999;52:180–4.
13. Bergmann M, Puskas Z, Kuchelmeister K. Subdural hematoma due to dural metastasis: case report and review of the literature. Clin Neurol Neurosurg 1992;94:235–40.
14. Beck J, Gralla J, Fung C, et al. Spinal cerebrospinal fluid leak as the cause of chronic subdural hematomas in nongeriatric patients. J Neurosurg 2014;121:1380–7.
15. Schreiber MA, Aoki N, Scott BG, et al. Determinants of mortality in patients with severe blunt head injury. Arch Surg 2002;137:285–90.
16. Mayer SA, Chong J. Critical care management of increased intracranial pressure. J Intensive Care Med 2002;17:55–67.
17. Badri S, Chen J, Barber J, et al. Mortality and long-term functional outcome associated with intracranial pressure after traumatic brain injury. Intensive Care Med 2012;38:1800–9.
18. Salvant JB Jr, Muizelaar JP. Changes in cerebral blood flow and metabolism related to the presence of subdural hematoma. Neurosurgery 1993;33(3):387–93.
19. Ersahin Y, Mutluer S. Posterior fossa extradural hematomas in children. Pediatr Neurosurg 1993;19:31–3.
20. Kortbeek JB, Al Turki SA, Ali J, et al. Advanced trauma life support, 8th edition, the evidence for change. J Trauma 2008;64:1638–50.

21. Stocchetti N, Furlan A, Volta F. Hypoxemia and arterial hypotension at the accident scene in head injury. J Trauma 1996;40:764–7.

22. National Clinical Guideline C. National Institutes for Health and clinical excellence: guidance. Head injury: triage, assessment, investigation and early management of head injury in children, young people and adults. London (United Kingdom): National Institute for Health and Care Excellence (UK); 2014.

23. Hodzovic I. Airway management disasters–lessons from the United Kingdom. Acta Clin Croat 2012;51:525–7.

24. Li J, Murphy-Lavoie H, Bugas C, et al. Complications of emergency intubation with and without paralysis. Am J Emerg Med 1999;17:141–3.

25. Tayal VS, Riggs RW, Marx JA, et al. Rapid-sequence intubation at an emergency medicine residency: success rate and adverse events during a two-year period. Acad Emerg Med 1999;6:31–7.

26. Bernard SA, Nguyen V, Cameron P, et al. Prehospital rapid sequence intubation improves functional outcome for patients with severe traumatic brain injury: a randomized controlled trial. Ann Surg 2010;252:959–65.

27. Peltoniemi MA, Hagelberg NM, Olkkola KT, et al. Ketamine: a review of clinical pharmacokinetics and pharmacodynamics in anesthesia and pain therapy. Clin Pharmacokinet 2016;55(9):1059–77.

28. Cohen L, Athaide V, Wickham ME, et al. The effect of ketamine on intracranial and cerebral perfusion pressure and health outcomes: a systematic review. Ann Emerg Med 2015;65:43–51.e42.

29. Gardner AE, Dannemiller FJ, Dean D. Intracranial cerebrospinal fluid pressure in man during ketamine anesthesia. Anesth Analg 1972;51:741–5.

30. Bruder EA, Ball IM, Ridi S, et al. Single induction dose of etomidate versus other induction agents for endotracheal intubation in critically ill patients. Cochrane Database Syst Rev 2015;(1):CD010225.

31. Gentry LR, Godersky JC, Thompson B, et al. Prospective comparative study of intermediate-field MR and CT in the evaluation of closed head trauma. AJR Am J Roentgenol 1988;150:673–82.

32. Frontera JA, Lewin JJ III, Rabinstein AA, et al. Guideline for reversal of antithrombotics in intracranial hemorrhage. Neurocrit Care 2016;24:6–46.

33. Wintzen AR, Tijssen JG. Subdural hematoma and oral anticoagulant therapy. Arch Neurol 1982;39:69–72.

34. Mattle H, Kohler S, Huber P, et al. Anticoagulation-related intracranial extracerebral haemorrhage. J Neurol Neurosurg Psychiatry 1989;52:829–37.

35. Narayan RK, Maas AI, Marshall LF, et al. Recombinant factor VIIa in traumatic intracerebral hemorrhage: results of a dose-escalation clinical trial. Neurosurgery 2008;62:776–86 [discussion: 786–8].

36. Feshchev I, Elran H, Salame K. Recombinant coagulation factor VIIa for rapid preoperative correction of warfarin-related coagulopathy in patients with acute subdural hematoma. Med Sci Monit 2002;8(12):CS98–100.

37. Garber ST, Sivakumar W, Schmidt RH. Neurosurgical complications of direct thrombin inhibitors–catastrophic hemorrhage after mild traumatic brain injury in a patient receiving dabigatran. J Neurosurg 2012;116:1093–6.

38. Reymond MA, Marbet G, Radu EW, et al. Aspirin as a risk factor for hemorrhage in patients with head injuries. Neurosurg Rev 1992;15:21–5.

39. Baharoglu MI, Cordonnier C, Salman RA, et al. Platelet transfusion versus standard care after acute stroke due to spontaneous cerebral haemorrhage associated with antiplatelet therapy (PATCH): a randomised, open-label, phase 3 trial. Lancet 2016;387(10038):2605–13.

40. Nishijima DK, Zehtabchi S, Berrong J, et al. Utility of platelet transfusion in adult patients with traumatic intracranial hemorrhage and preinjury antiplatelet use: a systematic review. J Trauma Acute Care Surg 2012;72:1658–63.

41. Mannucci PM, Remuzzi G, Pusineri F, et al. Deamino-8-d-arginine vasopressin shortens the bleeding time in uremia. N Engl J Med 1983;308:8–12.

42. Naidech AM, Maas MB, Levasseur-Franklin KE, et al. Desmopressin improves platelet activity in acute intracerebral hemorrhage. Stroke 2014;45:2451–3.

43. McMillian WD, Rogers FB. Management of prehospital antiplatelet and anticoagulant therapy in traumatic head injury: a review. J Trauma 2009;66:942–50.

44. Harhangi BS, Kompanje EJ, Leebeek FW, et al. Coagulation disorders after traumatic brain injury. Acta Neurochir 2008;150:165–75 [discussion: 175].

45. Allard CB, Scarpelini S, Rhind SG, et al. Abnormal coagulation tests are associated with progression of traumatic intracranial hemorrhage. J Trauma 2009;67:959–67.

46. Verweij BH, Muizelaar JP, Vinas FC. Hyperacute measurement of intracranial pressure, cerebral perfusion pressure, jugular venous oxygen saturation, and laser Doppler flowmetry, before and during removal of traumatic acute subdural hematoma. J Neurosurg 2001;95(4):569–72.

47. Stocchetti N, Maas AI, Chieregato A, et al. Hyperventilation in head injury: a review. Chest 2005;127:1812–27.

48. Coles JP, Minhas PS, Fryer TD, et al. Effect of hyperventilation on cerebral blood flow in traumatic head injury: clinical relevance and monitoring correlates. Crit Care Med 2002;30:1950–9.

49. Marion DW, Puccio A, Wisniewski SR, et al. Effect of hyperventilation on extracellular concentrations of glutamate, lactate, pyruvate, and local cerebral blood flow in patients with severe traumatic brain injury. Crit Care Med 2002;30:2619–25.

50. Muizelaar JP, Marmarou A, Ward JD, et al. Adverse effects of prolonged hyperventilation in patients with severe head injury: a randomized clinical trial. J Neurosurg 1991;75:731–9.

51. Obrist WD, Langfitt TW, Jaggi JL, et al. Cerebral blood flow and metabolism in comatose patients with acute head injury: relationship to intracranial hypertension. J Neurosurg 1984; 61(2):241–53.

52. Cruz J, Minoja G, Okuchi K. Improving clinical outcomes from acute subdural hematomas with the emergency preoperative administration of high doses of mannitol: a randomized trial. Neurosurgery 2001;49(4):864–71.

53. Andrews PJ, Sinclair HL, Rodriguez A, et al. Hypothermia for intracranial hypertension after traumatic brain injury. N Engl J Med 2015;373:2403–12.

54. Rabinstein AA, Chung SY, Rudzinski LA, et al. Seizures after evacuation of subdural hematomas: incidence, risk factors, and functional impact. J Neurosurg 2010;112:455–60.

55. Temkin NR, Dikmen SS, Wilensky AJ, et al. A randomized, double-blind study of phenytoin for the prevention of post-traumatic seizures. N Engl J Med 1990;323:497–502.

56. Schierhout G, Roberts I. Anti-epileptic drugs for preventing seizures following acute traumatic brain injury. Cochrane Database Syst Rev 2001;(4): CD000173.

57. Sabo RA, Hanigan WC, Aldag JC. Chronic subdural hematomas and seizures: the role of prophylactic anticonvulsive medication. Surg Neurol 1995; 43:579–82.

58. Kruer RM, Harris LH, Goodwin H, et al. Changing trends in the use of seizure prophylaxis after traumatic brain injury: a shift from phenytoin to levetiracetam. J Crit Care 2013;28:883.e9-13.

59. Inaba K, Menaker J, Branco BC, et al. A prospective multicenter comparison of levetiracetam versus phenytoin for early posttraumatic seizure prophylaxis. J Trauma acute Care Surg 2013;74:766–71 [discussion: 771–3].

60. Radic JA, Chou SH, Du R, et al. Levetiracetam versus phenytoin: a comparison of efficacy of seizure prophylaxis and adverse event risk following acute or subacute subdural hematoma diagnosis. Neurocrit Care 2014;21:228–37.

61. Edwards P, Arango M, Balica L, et al. Final results of MRC CRASH, a randomised placebo-controlled trial of intravenous corticosteroid in adults with head injury-outcomes at 6 months. Lancet 2005;365:1957–9.

62. Bratton SL, Chestnut RM, Ghajar J, et al. Guidelines for the management of severe traumatic brain injury. I. Blood pressure and oxygenation. J Neurotrauma 2007;24(Suppl 1):S7–13.

63. Bateman NT, Leach RM. ABC of oxygen. Acute oxygen therapy. BMJ 1998;317:798–801.

64. Lowe GJ, Ferguson ND. Lung-protective ventilation in neurosurgical patients. Curr Opin Crit Care 2006; 12:3–7.

65. Oddo M, Nduom E, Frangos S, et al. Acute lung injury is an independent risk factor for brain hypoxia after severe traumatic brain injury. Neurosurgery 2010;67:338–44.

66. McGuire G, Crossley D, Richards J, et al. Effects of varying levels of positive end-expiratory pressure on intracranial pressure and cerebral perfusion pressure. Crit Care Med 1997;25:1059–62.

67. Nemer SN, Caldeira JB, Santos RG, et al. Effects of positive end-expiratory pressure on brain tissue oxygen pressure of severe traumatic brain injury patients with acute respiratory distress syndrome: a pilot study. J Crit Care 2015;30:1263–6.

68. Busl KM, Ouyang B, Boland TA, et al. Prolonged mechanical ventilation is associated with pulmonary complications, increased length of stay, and unfavorable discharge destination among patients with subdural hematoma. J Neurosurg Anesthesiol 2015;27:31–6.

69. Lewis PM, Smielewski P, Rosenfeld JV, et al. Monitoring of the association between cerebral blood flow velocity and intracranial pressure. Acta Neurochir Suppl 2012;114:147–51.

70. Bouma GJ, Muizelaar JP, Bandoh K, et al. Blood pressure and intracranial pressure-volume dynamics in severe head injury: relationship with cerebral blood flow. J Neurosurg 1992;77:15–9.

71. Bouma GJ, Muizelaar JP. Cerebral blood flow, cerebral blood volume, and cerebrovascular reactivity after severe head injury. J Neurotrauma 1992;9(Suppl 1):S333–48.

72. Muizelaar JP, Ward JD, Marmarou A, et al. Cerebral blood flow and metabolism in severely head-injured children. Part 2: autoregulation. J Neurosurg 1989;71:72–6.

73. Juul N, Morris GF, Marshall SB, et al. Intracranial hypertension and cerebral perfusion pressure: influence on neurological deterioration and outcome in severe head injury. The executive committee of the International Selfotel Trial. J Neurosurg 2000; 92:1–6.

74. Andrews PJ, Sleeman DH, Statham PF, et al. Predicting recovery in patients suffering from traumatic brain injury by using admission variables and physiological data: a comparison between decision tree analysis and logistic regression. J Neurosurg 2002;97:326–36.

75. Anderson CS, Heeley E, Huang Y, et al. Rapid blood-pressure lowering in patients with acute intracerebral hemorrhage. N Engl J Med 2013; 368:2355–65.

76. Bratton SL, Chestnut RM, Ghajar J, et al. Guidelines for the management of severe traumatic brain injury. Ix. Cerebral perfusion thresholds. J Neurotrauma 2007;24(Suppl 1):S59–64.

77. Elf K, Nilsson P, Ronne-Engstrom E, et al. Cerebral perfusion pressure between 50 and 60 mm Hg may be beneficial in head-injured patients: a computerized secondary insult monitoring study. Neurosurgery 2005;56:962–71 [discussion: 962–71].

78. Jaeger M, Dengl M, Meixensberger J, et al. Effects of cerebrovascular pressure reactivity-guided optimization of cerebral perfusion pressure on brain tissue oxygenation after traumatic brain injury. Crit Care Med 2010;38:1343–7.

79. Grande PO. The "Lund concept" for the treatment of severe head trauma–physiological principles and clinical application. Intensive Care Med 2006;32:1475–84.

80. Busl KM, Raju M, Ouyang B, et al. Cardiac abnormalities in patients with acute subdural hemorrhage. Neurocrit Care 2013;19:176–82.

81. Barr J, Fraser GL, Puntillo K, et al. Clinical practice guidelines for the management of pain, agitation, and delirium in adult patients in the intensive care unit. Crit Care Med 2013;41:263–306.

82. Kelly DF, Goodale DB, Williams J, et al. Propofol in the treatment of moderate and severe head injury: a randomized, prospective double-blinded pilot trial. J Neurosurg 1999;90(6):1042–52.

83. Kam PC, Cardone D. Propofol infusion syndrome. Anaesthesia 2007;62(7):690–701.

84. Shafer A. Complications of sedation with midazolam in the intensive care unit and a comparison with other sedative regimens. Crit Care Med 1998;26(5):947–56.

85. Gu JW, Yang T, Kuang YQ, et al. Comparison of the safety and efficacy of propofol with midazolam for sedation of patients with severe traumatic brain injury: a meta-analysis. J Crit Care 2014;29:287–90.

86. Pajoumand M, Kufera JA, Bonds BW, et al. Dexmedetomidine as an adjunct for sedation in patients with traumatic brain injury. J Trauma Acute Care Surg 2016;81(2):345–51.

87. Venn M, Newman J, Grounds M. A phase II study to evaluate the efficacy of dexmedetomidine for sedation in the medical intensive care unit. Intensive Care Med 2003;29:201–7.

88. Jakob SM, Ruokonen E, Grounds RM, et al. Dexmedetomidine vs midazolam or propofol for sedation during prolonged mechanical ventilation: two randomized controlled trials. JAMA 2012;307: 1151–60.

89. Roberts DJ, Hall RI, Kramer AH, et al. Sedation for critically ill adults with severe traumatic brain injury: a systematic review of randomized controlled trials. Crit Care Med 2011;39:2743–51.

90. Cruz J. The first decade of continuous monitoring of jugular bulb oxyhemoglobin saturation: management strategies and clinical outcome. Crit Care Med 1998;26:344–51.

91. Bratton SL, Chestnut RM, Ghajar J, et al. Guidelines for the management of severe traumatic brain injury. X. Brain oxygen monitoring and thresholds. J Neurotrauma 2007;24(Suppl 1):S65–70.

92. Sheinberg M, Kanter MJ, Robertson CS, et al. Continuous monitoring of jugular venous oxygen saturation in head-injured patients. J Neurosurg 1992;76:212–7.

93. Maloney-Wilensky E, Gracias V, Itkin A, et al. Brain tissue oxygen and outcome after severe traumatic brain injury: a systematic review. Crit Care Med 2009;37:2057–63.

94. Pennings FA, Schuurman PR, van den Munckhof P, et al. Brain tissue oxygen pressure monitoring in awake patients during functional neurosurgery: the assessment of normal values. J Neurotrauma 2008;25:1173–7.

95. Stiefel MF, Spiotta A, Gracias VH, et al. Reduced mortality rate in patients with severe traumatic brain injury treated with brain tissue oxygen monitoring. J Neurosurg 2005;103:805–11.

96. Goodman JC, Robertson CS. Microdialysis: is it ready for prime time? Curr Opin Crit Care 2009; 15:110–7.

97. Hutchinson P, O'Phelan K. International multidisciplinary consensus conference on multimodality monitoring: cerebral metabolism. Neurocrit Care 2014;21(Suppl 2):S148–58.

98. Timofeev I, Carpenter KL, Nortje J, et al. Cerebral extracellular chemistry and outcome following traumatic brain injury: a microdialysis study of 223 patients. Brain 2011;134:484–94.

99. Andre C, de Freitas GR, Fukujima MM. Prevention of deep venous thrombosis and pulmonary embolism following stroke: a systematic review of published articles. Eur J Neurol 2007;14:21–32.

100. Greer DM, Funk SE, Reaven NL, et al. Impact of fever on outcome in patients with stroke and neurologic injury: a comprehensive meta-analysis. Stroke 2008;39:3029–35.

101. Diringer MN. Treatment of fever in the neurologic intensive care unit with a catheter-based heat exchange system. Crit Care Med 2004;32: 559–64.

102. Finfer S, Chittock DR, Su SY, et al. Intensive versus conventional glucose control in critically ill patients. N Engl J Med 2009;360:1283–97.

103. Oddo M, Schmidt JM, Carrerra E, et al. Impact of tight glycemic control on brain glucose levels after

severe brain injury: a microdialysis study. Crit Care Med 2008;36:3233–8.

104. Shackford SR, Zhuang J, Schmoker J. Intravenous fluid tonicity: effect on intracranial pressure, cerebral blood flow, and cerebral oxygen delivery in focal brain injury. J Neurosurg 1992;76(1):91–8.

105. Tommasino C, Moore S, Todd MM. Cerebral effects of isovolemic hemodilution with crystalloid or colloid solutions. Crit Care Med 1988;16(9):862–8.

106. Ertmer C, Aken H. Fluid therapy in patients with brain injury: what does physiology tell us? Crit Care 2014;18(2):119.

107. Clifton GL, Miller ER, Choi SC, et al. Fluid thresholds and outcome from severe brain injury. Crit Care Med 2002;30:739–45.

108. Badjatia N, Vespa P. Monitoring nutrition and glucose in acute brain injury. Neurocrit Care 2014;21(Suppl 2):S159–67.

109. Zarbock SD, Steinke D, Hatton J, et al. Successful enteral nutritional support in the neurocritical care unit. Neurocrit Care 2008;9:210–6.

110. Cook DJ, Reeve BK, Guyatt GH, et al. Stress ulcer prophylaxis in critically ill patients. Resolving discordant meta-analyses. JAMA 1996;275:308–14.

111. Misra UK, Kalita J, Pandey S, et al. Predictors of gastrointestinal bleeding in acute intracerebral haemorrhage. J Neurol Sci 2003;208:25–9.

112. Lasky MR, Metzler MH, Phillips JO. A prospective study of omeprazole suspension to prevent clinically significant gastrointestinal bleeding from stress ulcers in mechanically ventilated trauma patients. J Trauma 1998;44:527–33.

113. Tryba M. Prophylaxis of stress ulcer bleeding. A meta-analysis. J Clin Gastroenterol 1991;13(Suppl 2):S44–55.

Management of Recurrent Subdural Hematomas

Virendra R. Desai, MD*, Robert A. Scranton, MD, Gavin W. Britz, MD

KEYWORDS

- Subdural hematoma • Chronic subdural hematoma • Recurrent subdural hematoma
- Recurrent hematoma

KEY POINTS

- Subdural hematomas recur at a rate of 2% to 37% after surgical evacuation.
- Risk factors for recurrence include patient-related, radiologic, and surgical risk factors; patient-related risk factors include alcoholism, seizure disorders, and history of ventriculoperitoneal shunt placement. Most studies have shown age, sex, hypertension, anticoagulant or antiplatelet usage, and cause of hematoma (trauma, after craniotomy, and so forth) have no impact on recurrence.
- Radiologic risk factors include preoperative appearance of bilateral hematomas, greater midline shift, heterogeneous hematomas (layered or multi-loculated), and more acute-appearing, hyperdense hematomas. Postoperative risk factors include poor brain reexpansion and presence of a significant amount of subdural air.
- Surgical risk factors include lack of or poor postoperative closed-system drainage.
- Most recurrent subdural hematomas can be managed successfully via burr hole craniostomy and postoperative closed-system drainage; refractory hematomas may require craniotomy, subdural-peritoneal shunt placement, placement of subdural catheter connected to Rickham reservoir with serial tapping, endoscopic removal, continuous postoperative irrigation and drainage, or injection of isotonic fluid into the ventricular space to promote brain reexpansion.

INTRODUCTION

Chronic subdural hematomas are a common pathologic condition, especially of the elderly. These lesions can at times be managed medically without surgical intervention if they are small with minimal mass effect and if the lesions are not significantly symptomatic. At other times, they require surgical intervention for symptomatic relief and/or avoiding mortality.

Multiple surgical methods have been described, including bedside twist drill trephination, formal burr hole trephination, craniotomy with resection of neomembranes, and subdural-peritoneal shunt placement.[1–10] All of these techniques may or may not involve irrigation of the subdural space,

and both burr hole and craniotomy techniques may or may not involve temporary postoperative closed-system drainage. Single or double burr hole evacuation with or without postoperative closed-system drainage has been proven to successfully treat these lesions and is the most common method used.[1–4,7,8,10–12]

However, hematomas can recur. Recurrence can be defined as any radiologic recurrence, which can be asymptomatic, mild to moderately symptomatic recurrence requiring medical management, or severely symptomatic recurrence requiring surgical evacuation.[12,13] The rate of clinically significant recurrence that requires surgical evacuation ranges from 7.0% to 26.5% after initial burr hole evacuation with or without postoperative

Department of Neurosurgery, Houston Methodist Hospital, 6565 Fannin Street, Houston, TX 77030, USA
* Corresponding author.
E-mail address: vrdesai@houstonmethodist.org

Neurosurg Clin N Am 28 (2017) 279–286
http://dx.doi.org/10.1016/j.nec.2016.11.010
1042-3680/17/© 2016 Elsevier Inc. All rights reserved.

closed-system drainage.[1–3,12] Over all types of initial operations, the rate ranges from 2% to 37%.[4,10,13] The average time from initial operation to the second one ranges from 6 days to 3.5 weeks after the first operation.[13–15]

PATIENT-SPECIFIC RISK FACTORS

Given the high recurrence rate after subdural hematoma evacuation, a thorough understanding of risk factors leading to such recurrence is paramount. Risk factors for subdural hematoma recurrence can be split into 3 groups: first, patient factors, such as age, sex, comorbidities, alcohol abuse, anticoagulant and/or antiplatelet use, brain atrophy, bleeding tendency, or intracranial hypotension; second, subdural hematoma factors, such as hematoma size and location, presence of membranes, and acute versus chronic; and third, surgical factors, such as timing of surgery, single burr hole versus multiple burr holes versus craniotomy, irrigation, and drainage.[2,5–9]

Commonly associated risk factors are chronic alcoholism; well-known predisposing factors include shunt procedures leading to intracranial hypotension (**Fig. 1**), seizure disorders, and impaired coagulation.[5,11,12,16] Oishi and colleagues[5] performed a retrospective review of 116 patients and found in their recurrence group a significantly lower incidence of head injury and significantly lower interval from symptom onset to hospitalization. Jung and colleagues[10] performed a retrospective review of 182 patients and found a significant clinical history risk factor was hemiparesis. Diabetes mellitus trends toward increased recurrence in some studies[3]; however, it has no significance in others.[1] Yamamoto and colleagues[16] found a higher recurrence rate in the absence of diabetes mellitus.

Clearly, further studies are needed to delineate medical comorbidities that predispose to recurrence.

Most studies have found no difference in recurrence rate in terms of age, sex, hypertension, heart

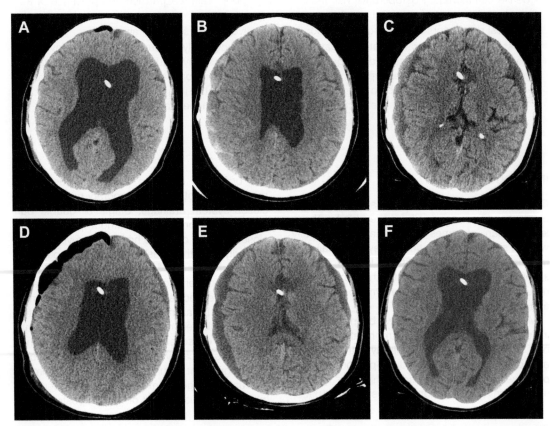

Fig. 1. (*A*) Immediate postoperative computed tomography scan after ventriculoperitoneal shunt placement. (*B*) Delayed presentation of bilateral subdural hematomas, trabecular or multi-loculated type on the right. (*C*) After waiting for a short number of days, the subdural hematoma grew more hypodense, appearing as the separated or layered type. The patient then underwent burr hole evacuation. (*D*) Immediately after burr hole evacuation, note the poor brain reexpansion and significant subdural air. (*E*) Recurrence of hematoma, appearing as the homogeneous, hypodense type. (*F*) Repeat burr hole evacuation lead to complete resolution.

disease, antiplatelet or anticoagulant use, or cause of hematoma (trauma vs unknown vs after craniotomy).[3,6,10]

RADIOLOGIC RISK FACTORS

Radiographic factors involved in postoperative recurrence rate include hematoma location in convexity versus skull base; internal architecture as proposed by Nakaguchi and colleagues[17] (homogenous density [high, low, or isodense], laminar [mixed density], separated [known as layered] including gradation subtype, and trabecular [multi-loculated] [see **Fig. 1**]); unilateral versus bilateral; midline shift; width of subdural space; subdural hematoma volume; and presence of air.[1,3,5,6,10]

Poor reexpansion of the brain after hematoma evacuation has been extensively studied as a predisposing factor for recurrence (see **Fig. 1**D).[1,5,18,19] Mori and Maeda[1] analyzed 500 cases of burr hole evacuation of subdural hematomas with closed-system drainage and found that brain reexpansion at 1 week occurred in 45% of patients with recurrence and 55% without recurrence (P<.001). They identified age greater than 70 years, preexisting cerebral infarction, and persistent subdural air as significant correlates of poor brain reexpansion (P<.001).[1] The presence of substantial subdural air hinders reduction of the cavity created by hematoma evacuation and increases the recurrence rate (see **Fig. 1**D).[5,6,20]

Poor brain reexpansion is related to high brain surface elastance, which is correlated with greater age, fibrous organization of subdural neomembranes, and impaired cerebral blood flow.[18,19] Fukuhara and colleagues[18] analyzed the relationship between brain surface elastance and hematoma recurrence by evacuating hematomas via burr holes, placing a Muller ophthalmodynamometer on the brain surface and compressing the brain to 5 mm Hg. They then measured the depth required to reach this pressure (which they defined as the brain elastance). They found that those who had a subdural space greater than 3 mm 1 month postoperatively, relative to those with less than 3 mm, had a significantly higher brain surface elastance (ie, their brain could be compressed to a greater depth until 5 mm Hg pressure was reached). They found some correlation between age and elastance, no correlation between volume of hematoma and elastance, and a tendency for those with high-density hematomas and more symptomatic patients (drowsy and/or neurologic deficit or worse) to be correlated with elastance, although this correlation was nonsignificant. They suggest that high brain

elastance leads to poor brain reexpansion and can predispose to recurrence; thus, measuring brain elastance can be a tool to help predict recurrence.[18]

Markwalder and colleagues[19] studied the relationship between subdural pressure, intracranial pressure, and brain reexpansion postoperatively and found that brain reexpansion was promoted by higher subdural (>25 cm H_2O) and intracranial pressures and inhibited by a thick fibrotic neomembrane.

With regard to the hematoma's internal architecture, the recurrence rate is generally lower in the homogeneous type and significantly higher in the separated type, including gradation subtype (see **Fig. 1**C, E). Within homogeneous types, the recurrence rate was significantly lower in the low-density subtype relative to other types.[6,21] Oishi and colleagues[5] found a higher rate of recurrence in patients who had any component of hyperintensity on preoperative computed tomography (CT) scan, suggesting a more acute hematoma, 15.6% versus 1.7% (see **Fig. 1**B). The investigators suggest this may be an indication of vulnerable capillaries within a neomembrane, which forms secondary to inflammation induced by the blood itself. Nakaguchi and colleagues[17] theorize that this may be secondary to the limited organization of the younger hematoma (immature fibrosis of the neomembranes or trabeculae). Oishi and colleagues[5] suggest postponing surgical evacuation, unless emergent, until the hematoma appears isodense or hypodense on CT scan. (However, it must be noted that these cases were performed with single burr hole surgery; thus, any acute, clotted blood may have not been evacuated.)

Subdural hematomas can recur ipsilaterally or contralaterally. Thin subdural hematomas on the contralateral side are a high risk of recurrence contralaterally.[1] Bilateral hematomas are significant risk factors for recurrence.[3,10,21]

It was also significantly higher with greater midline shift (>5 mm in one study, >10 mm in another) and the presence of acute clots (which were only seen postoperatively in cranial base subdural hematomas).[6,10] There is a higher correlation of recurrence with maximum width of subdural space greater than 10 mm.[6,20]

Stanisic and colleagues[22] found that preoperative subdural hematoma volume of less than 115 mL and postoperative volume of less than 80 mL were strongly correlated with no recurrence (94.4% and 97.4% respectively). On the other hand, Huang and colleagues[23] found no significance of hematoma volume on recurrence rate.

SURGICAL RISK FACTORS

As noted previously, there are multiple operative techniques currently used to evacuate chronic subdural hematomas. Weigel and colleagues[8] did a systematic review of literature and compared multiple different techniques, including twist drill craniostomy (hole diameter up to 5 mm), burr hole craniostomy (hole diameter up to 30 mm), and larger openings, such as craniotomies. They found most studies used one of these 3 methods with or without irrigation and with or without postoperative closed-system drainage. Craniotomies had a morbidity rate of 12.3%, mortality rate of 4.6%, and recurrence rate of 10.8%. In contrast, twist drill craniostomies and burr hole craniostomies, respectively, had a morbidity rate of 3.0% and 3.8%, mortality rate of 2.9% and 2.7%, and recurrence rate of 33.0% and 12.1%. The differences in mortality rates were not significant, whereas craniotomy techniques had significantly higher morbidity than twist drill or burr hole techniques; recurrence rates were significantly lower in craniotomy and burr hole techniques relative to twist drill craniostomy techniques.[8,24] It is important to note that the studies comparing these techniques are not controlled randomized trials and, thus, the patients selected for craniotomy may have been those suspected to have a higher morbidity or probability of recurrence.[8]

Commonly, a closed-system drainage tube is used several days postoperatively. Markwalder and Seiler[25] performed a case series of 21 patients and found progressive clinical improvement when closed-system drainage was used.[7] Wakai and colleagues[2] did a prospective study on 38 patients and also found a lower recurrence rate when closed-system drainage used: 33% versus 5%.[7] Santarius and colleagues[26] did a randomized controlled trial evaluating recurrence rate of subdural hematoma after evacuation with and without drain placement. The trial was stopped early because of a significant benefit of drain placement with 9.3% recurrence with drain and 24% without. Weigel and colleagues[8] also compared twist drill craniostomy with and without drainage and found a significantly lower recurrence rate with drainage.

Kwon and colleagues[11] analyzed 175 patients who underwent burr hole trephination with closed-system drainage for 5 days and found a significantly higher recurrence rate in patients who had less than 200 mL of drainage volume postoperatively relative to those who had more than 200 mL.

Jung and colleagues[10] found no difference in recurrence rate with one versus 2 burr holes or location of drainage tube (none, frontal, occipital, or parietal). Others, on the other hand, have found a significantly lower recurrence rate when the tip of the drainage tube was in a frontal position as opposed to temporal, occipital, or parietal.[8,27]

Commonly, patients are kept in a flat, supine position postoperatively to decrease the recurrence rate. Abouzari and colleagues[12] evaluated 84 patients who underwent single burr hole trephination for evacuation and irrigation of chronic traumatic subdural hematoma and postoperative closed-system drainage. They randomly assigned the patients into 2 groups: one that was placed in a supine, flat position for 3 days postoperatively and the other placed with the head of the bed elevated to 30° to 40° for the same time frame. They defined recurrence via clinical or radiologic criteria and found a significantly higher rate in those patients sitting with the head elevated relative to those kept flat. However, only one of these recurrences in the former group was significant enough to require reoperation. There were no significant differences in terms of complications from lying flat, such as atelectasis and/or pneumonia.[12] On the other hand, Nakajima and colleagues[28] found no difference in recurrence rates with the same trial design as Abouzari and colleagues.[12]

Some surgeons stress irrigation of the subdural space to remove as much subdural fluid and/or acute clots as possible and replace it with saline or lactated Ringer solution. Lee and colleagues[29] compared 2 groups retrospectively: one in which a subdural catheter was placed via burr hole trephination and saline instilled until the fluid exuded clear and a second group in which a subdural catheter was placed but no irrigation was performed. Both groups underwent postoperative closed-system drainage for at least 48 hours. These investigators found a significantly lower rate of recurrence with irrigation than without in a group who underwent burr hole craniostomy and postoperative closed-system drainage.[29]

Ishibasi and colleagues[30] retrospectively compared a group with burr hole drainage only (in which a single burr hole was placed with postoperative closed-system drainage) to a group with burr hole drainage with irrigation and found a significantly higher recurrence rate in the drainage only group (10.3% vs 2.9%).

On the other hand, Okada and colleagues[31] had the opposite results. These investigators compared 2 groups: irrigation and drainage. The irrigation group had a subdural catheter placed via a burr hole and the hematoma was irrigated until the fluid exuded was clear. The drainage group had a catheter placed in the subdural space and was drained at a slow rate postoperatively. The drainage group had a significantly lower rate of recurrence (5% vs 25%).[31] Kuroki and colleagues[32] also compared 2 groups, one in which a subdural catheter was placed without irrigation and taking care not to introduce air into the subdural cavity and another group in which the subdural space was irrigated and then a catheter was placed (the subdural space was filled with saline on closure with the burr hole at the highest point to introduce as little air as possible). The drainage group without irrigation had a significantly lower rate of recurrence (1.8% vs 11.1%), lower duration of drainage, and faster disappearance of hematoma. Given the conflicting results of irrigation, a randomized controlled trial would be necessary to further elucidate the role of intraoperative irrigation on recurrence rates.

Ram and colleagues[33] and Hennig and Kloster[34] evaluated the significance of postoperative continuous inflow and outflow irrigation and drainage. Ram and colleagues[33] found a significantly lower rate of recurrence with continuous postoperative irrigation. Hennig and Kloster[34] compared 4 groups: burr hole craniostomy with continuous inflow and outflow drainage postoperatively for up to 48 hours, burr hole craniostomy with intraoperative irrigation and postoperative closed-system drainage, burr hole craniostomy with intraoperative irrigation only, and craniotomy. They found a significantly lower rate of recurrence in the continuous drainage group, 2.6%, relative to the other groups (23.8%, 32.6%, 44.4%, respectively).[34] These findings suggest that although intraoperative irrigation has an uncertain impact on recurrence, postoperative continuous irrigation and drainage can lower it.

FLUID CHARACTERISTICS

Given the uncertain role of irrigation, several investigators have analyzed the subdural fluid itself to understand its origin and its composition. Kwon and colleagues[11] sought to evaluate where the fluid from recurrent subdural hematomas comes from by intravenously injecting several patients with radioactive tracer immediately after surgery and measuring tracer amount in plasma, cerebrospinal fluid (CSF), and subdural drainage. They found that the tracer amounts were similar in plasma and subdural drainage with very limited detection in CSF. The investigators, therefore, propose that most of the recurrent subdural fluid stems from plasma exudation between gap junctions between endothelial cells of subdural neomembranes.[11]

As noted previously, Kwon and colleagues[11] found a higher recurrence rate when the postoperative drainage amount was less than 200 mL. They

theorize that this may be due to the presence of anticlotting factors in the subdural fluid that open gap junctions between endothelial cells in the subdural neomembrane, which may otherwise be closed in the short-term by thrombi and other factors. When higher postoperative drainage amounts occur, this implied increased plasma exudation; this intrinsic irrigation would lead to further dilution of anticlotting factors.[11] This theory is concordant with the finding that higher recurrence rates are found with high- or mixed-density postoperative subdural fluid relative to lower-density fluid, as higher density signifies more acute clot formation, which could temporarily obstruct the gap junctions between endothelial cells.[6,11] When the hematomas are evacuated, the intraluminal pressure within the endothelial cells drops, leading to a gradual reduction in the gap junctions between endothelial cells and thereby a gradual reduction in membrane permeability.[11]

Frati and colleagues[35] found a higher concentration of the inflammatory cytokines interleukin 6 and interleukin 8 in the subdural fluid for recurrent hematomas. These investigators suggest administering antiinflammatory medication postoperatively may reduce the risk of recurrence.

Unterhofer and colleagues[36] performed a prospective randomized trial comparing recurrence rates with and without opening of the internal hematoma membranes and found no difference in recurrence rates. Weigel and colleagues[8] also note that although the craniotomy technique involves resection of the hematoma membranes, the burr hole technique simply involves removal of hematoma fluid. These investigators infer that because both techniques have similar recurrence rates, the hematoma fluid itself is responsible for recurrence rather than the neomembranes. This theory is supported by multiple publications that demonstrate the large concentration of vasoactive mediators, such as vascular endothelial growth factor, inflammatory mediators, and fibrinolytic factors.[8,29]

SURGICAL MANAGEMENT

Management of a recurrent subdural hematoma has not been well defined. Weigel and colleagues[8] report 20 publications that evaluated treatment of recurrences after burr hole craniostomy and found 85% were treated successfully with the same procedure as initially performed, whereas 14% underwent craniotomy and 1% died.[2,19,25,33,37–52] They found 7 publications concerning management of recurrence after twist drill craniostomy and found 70% treated successfully after the same procedure a second or third time, 24% had burr hole craniostomies performed, and 6% had craniotomy performed.[8,47,53–58] They found no studies concerning management of recurrence after craniotomy.[8] As noted earlier, craniotomies have a significantly higher morbidity rate relative to twist drill and burr hole techniques; thus, they recommend twist drill or burr hole trephination over craniotomy even for recurrences. Based on their results, they make the following type C recommendations: burr hole craniostomy is more effective in treating recurrent hematoma than twist drill craniostomy, and craniotomy should be considered the last treatment option.[8]

Although many recurrences can be successfully treated via repeat burr hole craniostomy, some will require added measures to ensure no recurrence, such as craniotomy, closed-system drainage, postoperative continuous irrigation and drainage, shunt placement, and so forth. Cenic and colleagues[7] performed a national survey of Canadian neurosurgeons on their management of initial and recurrent subdural hematomas and found a higher use of more invasive operations, such as craniotomy and subdural-peritoneal shunt for recurrence, and lower use of twist drill or single burr hole surgery for recurrence, as would be expected. They found 2-burr hole surgery and craniotomy as the preferred methods in recurrence.

Subdural-peritoneal drainage may be a reasonable option for refractory recurrent subdural hematomas.[7,59,60]

Laumer and colleagues[61] performed a prospective study on 144 patients, comparing recurrence rates after subdural hematoma evacuation with external closed-system drainage, with aspiration and irrigation but no postoperative drainage, and with permanent subdural drain placement with subcutaneous reservoir. The permanent subdural drain was placed via a multi-perforated catheter placed into the subdural space from a frontoparietal burr hole and connected to a Rickham reservoir. Although the hematoma recurrence rates were similar between all 3 groups, the reoperation rates were 4-fold lower for the permanent drain/subcutaneous reservoir group. This finding was because any symptomatic recurrence confirmed by CT scan was first subjected to aspiration via Rickham reservoir tapping and aspiration at bedside before surgery was considered.[61]

Hellwig and colleagues[41] described a method of endoscopic removal of recurrent subdural hematoma via a small burr hole.

Robinson,[46] realizing how poor brain reexpansion predisposes to recurrence, did a study on injecting lactated Ringer solution into the CSF, either via lumbar puncture or directly into the anterior horn of the lateral ventricle, to promote brain reexpansion. He found a benefit in this technique for more symptomatic hematomas, bilateral hematomas, and the elderly.

Given the aforementioned findings, although a repeat burr hole craniostomy may successfully treat most recurrences, refractory subdural hematomas may require added measures. Several available options to the neurosurgeon exist, including craniotomy, subdural-peritoneal drainage, placement of subdural catheter connected to Rickham reservoir for serial tapping, endoscopic evacuation, or injecting isotonic fluid into the CSF to promote brain expansion.

SUMMARY

Subdural hematomas have a recurrence rate of 2% to 37% after surgical evacuation. Risk factors for recurrence are split into 3 groups: patient related, radiologic, and surgical. Patient-related risk factors include chronic alcoholism, seizure disorders, and history of ventriculoperitoneal shunt. The impact of diabetes mellitus is controversial; most studies suggest age, sex, hypertension, cardiac disease, and use of anticoagulants or antiplatelets do not influence the recurrence rate. Radiologic risk factors include preoperative appearance of heterogeneous hematoma or higher-density hematoma, greater midline shift, and bilateral hematomas or postoperative appearance of poor brain reexpansion or greater subdural air. Surgical risk factors include the use of twist drill craniostomy as opposed to burr hole craniostomy or craniotomy, although craniotomies predispose to higher morbidity rates. Other surgical risk factors include lack of or poor postoperative closed-system drainage. The impact of intraoperative irrigation and postoperative patient position (flat vs upright) is controversial. Many recurrent hematomas can be successfully managed by repeat burr hole craniostomy with postoperative closed-system drainage. Some refractory hematomas may require additional measures, and available options include craniotomy, subdural-peritoneal shunting, placement of subdural catheter connected to Rickham reservoir for serial tapping, endoscopic evacuation, or injection of isotonic fluid into the ventricular space to promote brain expansion.

REFERENCES

1. Mori K, Maeda M. Surgical treatment of chronic subdural hematoma in 500 consecutive cases: clinical characteristics, surgical outcome, complications, and recurrence rate. Neurol Med Chir (Tokyo) 2001;41:371–81.

2. Wakai S, Hashimoto K, Watanabe N, et al. Efficacy of closed-system drainage in treating chronic subdural hematoma: a prospective comparative study. Neurosurgery 1990;26(5):771–3.

3. Torihashi K, Sadamasa N, Yoshida K, et al. Independent predictors for recurrence of chronic subdural hematoma: a review of 343 consecutive surgical cases. Neurosurgery 2008;63(6):1125–9.

4. Schwarz F, Loos F, Dunisch P, et al. Risk factors for reoperation after initial burr hole trephination in chronic subdural hematomas. Clin Neurol Neurosurg 2015;138:66–71.

5. Oishi M, Toyama M, Tamatani S, et al. Clinical factors of recurrent chronic subdural hematoma. Neurol Med Chir (Tokyo) 2001;41:382–6.

6. Stanisic M, Lund-Johansen M, Mahesparan R. Treatment of chronic subdural hematoma by burr-hole craniostomy in adults: influence of some factors on postoperative recurrence. Acta Neurochir (Wien) 2005;147:1249–57.

7. Cenic A, Bhandari M, Reddy K. Management of chronic subdural hematoma: a national survey and literature review. Can J Neurol Sci 2005;32(4):501–6.

8. Weigel R, Schmiedek P, Krauss JK. Outcome of contemporary surgery for chronic subdural haematoma: evidence based review. J Neurol Neurosurg Psychiatry 2003;74:937–43.

9. Markwalder TM. Chronic subdural hematomas: a review. J Neurosurg 1981;54:637–45.

10. Jung YG, Jung NY, Kim E. Independent predictors for recurrence of chronic subdural hematoma. J Korean Neurosurg Soc 2015;57(4):266–70.

11. Kwon TH, Park YK, Lim DJ, et al. Chronic subdural hematoma: evaluation of the clinical significance of postoperative drainage volume. J Neurosurg 2000; 93:796–9.

12. Abouzari M, Rashidi A, Rezaii J, et al. The role of postoperative patient posture in the recurrence of traumatic chronic subdural hematoma after burr-hole surgery. Neurosurgery 2007;61:794–7.

13. Desai V, Sparrow II, Grossman R. Incidence of intracranial hemorrhage after a cranial operation. Cureus 2016;8(5):e616.

14. Komotar RJ, Starke RM, Connolly ES. The role of drain placement following chronic subdural hematoma evacuation. Neurosurgery 2010;66(2): N15–6.

15. Gokmen M, Sucu HK, Ergin A, et al. Randomized comparative study of burr-hole craniostomy versus twist drill craniostomy: surgical management of unilateral hemispheric chronic subdural hematomas. Zentralbl Neurochir 2008;69(3):129–33.

16. Yamamoto H, Hirashima Y, Hamada H, et al. Independent predictors of recurrence of chronic subdural hematoma: results of multivariate analysis performed using a logistic regression model. J Neurosurg 2003;98(6):1217–21.

17. Nakaguchi H, Tanishama T, Yoshimasu N. Factors in the natural history of chronic subdural hematomas that influence their postoperative recurrence. J Neurosurg 2001;95(2):256–62.

18. Fukuhara T, Gotoh M, Asari S, et al. The relationship between brain surface elastance and brain reexpansion after evacuation of chronic subdural hematoma. Surg Neurol 1996;45:570–4.

19. Markwalder TM, Steinsiepe KF, Rohner M, et al. The course of chronic subdural hematomas after burr-hole craniostomy and closed-system drainage. J Neurosurg 1981;55:390–6.

20. Ohba S, Kinoshita Y, Nakagawa T, et al. The risk factors for recurrence of chronic subdural hematoma. Neurosurg Rev 2013;36(1):145–50.

21. Song DH, Kim YS, Chun HJ, et al. The predicting factors for recurrence of chronic subdural hematoma treated with burr hole and drainage. Korean J Neurotrauma 2014;10(2):41–8.

22. Stanisic M, Hald J, Rasmussen IA, et al. Volume and densities of chronic subdural haematoma obtained from CT imaging as predictors of postoperative recurrence: a prospective study of 107 operated patients. Acta Neurochir (Wien) 2013; 155(2):323–33.

23. Huang YH, Lin WC, Lu CH, et al. Volume of chronic subdural haematoma: is it one of the radiographic factors related to recurrence? Injury 2014;45(9):1327–31.

24. Schulz W, Saballus R, Flugel R, et al. Chronic subdural hematoma. A comparison of bore hole trepanation and craniotomy. Zentralbl Neurochir 1988;49:280–9.

25. Markwalder TM, Seiler RW. Chronic subdural hematomas: to drain or not to drain? Neurosurgery 1985; 16:185–8.

26. Santarius T, Kirkpatrick PJ, Ganesan D, et al. Use of drains versus no drains after burr-hole evacuation of chronic subdural haematoma: a randomized controlled trial. Lancet 2009;374(9695):1067–73.

27. Nakaguchi H, Tanishima T, Yoshimasu N. Relationship between drainage catheter location and postoperative recurrence of chronic subdural hematoma after burr-hole irrigation and closed-system drainage. J Neurosurg 2000;93(5):791–5.

28. Nakajima H, Yasui T, Nishikawa M, et al. The role of postoperative patient posture in the recurrence of chronic subdural hematoma: a prospective randomized trial. Surg Neurol 2002;58:385–7.

29. Lee C, Park DS, Song SW, et al. Effect of intraoperative saline irrigation during burr hole surgery on the recurrence for chronic subdural hematomas. The Nerve 2015;1(1):26–9. Available online at: http://thenerve.net/journal/view.php?doi=10.21129/nerve.2015.1.1.26.

30. Ishibasi A, Yokokura Y, Adachi H. A comparative study of treatments for chronic subdural hematoma: burr hole drainage versus burr hole drainage with irrigation. Kurume Med J 2011;58:35–9.

31. Okada Y, Akai T, Okamoto K, et al. A comparative study of the treatment of chronic subdural hematoma-burr hole drainage versus burr hole irrigation. Surg Neurol 2002;57:405–9.

32. Kuroki T, Katsume M, Harada N, et al. Strict closed-system drainage for treating chronic subdural haematoma. Acta Neurochir (Wien) 2001;143:1041–4.

33. Ram Z, Hadani M, Sahar A, et al. Continuous irrigation-drainage of the subdural space for the treatment of chronic subdural hematoma. A prospective clinical trial. Acta Neurochir 1993;120:40–3.

34. Hennig R, Kloster R. Burr hole evacuation of chronic subdural haematomas followed by continuous inflow and outflow irrigation. Acta Neurochir 1999;141: 171–6.

35. Frati A, Salvati M, Mainiero F, et al. Inflammation markers and risk factors for recurrence in 35 patients with a posttraumatic chronic subdural hematoma: a prospective study. J Neurosurg 2004; 100(1):24–32.

36. Unterhofer C, Freyschlag CF, Thome C, et al. Opening the internal hematoma membrane does not alter the recurrence rate of chronic subdural hematomas: a prospective randomized trial. World Neurosurg 2016;92:31–6.

37. Benzel EC, Bridges RM, Hadden TA, et al. The single burr hole technique for the evacuation of nonacute subdural hematomas. J Trauma 1994;36: 190–4.

38. Choudhury AR. Avoidable factors that contribute to complications in the surgical treatment of chronic subdural haematoma. Acta Neurochir (Wien) 1994; 129(1–2):15–9.

39. Drapkin AJ. Chronic subdural hematoma: pathophysiological basis for treatment. Br J Neurosurg 1991;5:467–73.

40. Harders A, Eggert HR, Weigel K. Treatment of chronic subdural hematoma by closed external drainage. Neurochirurgia (Stuttg) 1982;25:147–52.

41. Hellwig D, Kuhn TJ, Bauer BL, et al. Endoscopic treatment of septated chronic subdural hematoma. Surg Neurol 1996;45:272–7.

42. Kotwica Z, Brzezinski J. Chronic subdural haematoma treated by burr holes and closed system drainage: personal experience in 131 patients. Br J Neurosurg 1991;5:461–5.

43. Krupp WF, Jans PJ. Treatment of chronic subdural haematoma with burr-hole craniostomy and closed drainage. Br J Neurosurg 1995;9:619–27.

44. Kuroki T, Matsumoto M, Kushida T, et al. Nontraumatic subdural hematoma secondary to dural metastasis of lung cancer: case report and review of the literature. No Shinkei Geka 1994;22:857–62.

45. Piotrowski WP, Krombholz-Reindl MA. Surgical outcome in chronic subdural hematoma. Unfallchirurgie 1996;22:110–6.

46. Robinson RG. Chronic subdural hematoma: surgical management in 133 patients. J Neurosurg 1984;61: 263–8.

47. Smely C, Madlinger A, Scheremet R. Chronic subdural haematoma – a comparison of two different treatment modalities. Acta Neurochir (Wien) 1997; 139:818–25.

48. Spallone A, Giuffre R, Gagliardi FM, et al. Chronic subdural hematoma in extremely aged patients. Eur Neurol 1989;29(1):18–22.

49. Van Havenbergh T, van Calenbergh F, Goffin J, et al. Outcome of chronic subdural haematoma: analysis of prognostic factors. Br J Neurosurg 1996;10:35–9.

50. Weir BK. Results of burr hole and open or closed suction drainage for chronic subdural hematomas in adults. Can J Neurol Sci 1983;10:22–6.

51. Weisse A, Berney J. Chronic subdural haematomas. Results of a closed drainage method in adults. Acta Neurochir (Wien) 1994;127:37–40.

52. Yoshimoto Y, Kwak S. Frontal small craniostomy and irrigation for treatment of chronic subdural haematoma. Br J Neurosurg 1997;11:150–1.

53. Camel M, Grubb RL. Treatment of chronic subdural hematoma by twist-drill craniotomy with continuous catheter drainage. J Neurosurg 1986;65:183–7.

54. Aoki N. Subdural tapping and irrigation for the treatment of chronic subdural hematoma in adults. Neurosurgery 1984;14:545–8.

55. Aoki N. A new therapeutic method for chronic subdural hematoma in adults: replacement of the hematoma with oxygen via percutaneous subdural tapping. Surg Neurol 1992;38:253–6.

56. Carlton CK, Saunders RL. Twist drill craniostomy and closed system drainage of chronic and subacute subdural hematomas. Neurosurgery 1983; 13:153–9.

57. Reinges MH, Hasselberg I, Rohde V, et al. Prospective analysis of bedside percutaneous subdural tapping for the treatment of chronic subdural haematoma in adults. J Neurol Neurosurg Psychiatry 2000;69:40–7.

58. Rychlicki F, Rechionni MA, Burchianti M, et al. Percutaneous twist-drill craniostomy for the treatment of chronic subdural haematoma. Acta Neurochir (Wien) 1991;113:38–41.

59. Probst C. Peritoneal drainage of chronic subdural hematomas in older patients. J Neurosurg 1988;68: 908–11.

60. Alvarez-Pinzon A, Stein AA, Valerio JE, et al. Is subdural peritoneal shunt placement an effective tool for the management of recurrent/chronic subdural hematoma? Cureus 2016;8(5):e613.

61. Laumer R, Schramm J, Leykauf K. Implantation of a reservoir for recurrent subdural hematoma drainage. Neurosurgery 1989;25(6):991–6.

Perioperative Management of Anticoagulation

Daipayan Guha, MD[a],
R. Loch Macdonald, MD, PhD, FRCSC[a,b,*]

KEYWORDS

- Subdural hematoma • Anticoagulation • Antiplatelet • Bleeding • Thrombosis

KEY POINTS

- Antithrombotic drugs should be reversed emergently in all patients with chronic subdural hematomas (SDHs) who require urgent surgery; if surgery can be delayed, it is less certain whether to do this or to wait for spontaneous recovery from anticoagulation.
- There are no data to guide practitioners on whether or not to reverse antiplatelet drugs.
- Appropriate laboratory monitoring should guide the adequacy of reversal for all agents.
- Postoperative resumption of anticoagulant and antiplatelet drugs should be guided by a thorough and individualized assessment of hemorrhagic and thromboembolic risk.

INTRODUCTION

The use of antithrombotic agents, either antiplatelet or anticoagulant drugs, is expanding with a progressive rise in prevalence of patients with atherosclerotic risk factors as well as thrombogenic cardiac arrhythmias typically seen in the elderly.[1,2] There is strong evidence for short-term dual-antiplatelet therapy as the standard of care for patients with acute coronary syndromes[3,4] and oral anticoagulation in patients with atrial fibrillation at high risk of thromboembolism.[5]

Antiplatelet and anticoagulant drugs are known to predispose to the development of both acute and chronic SDHs.[6,7] These may occur in a dose-dependent manner; 1 series of patients on warfarin found an increase in subdural hemorrhage risk by more than 7-fold, with an increase in prothrombin ratio from 2.0 to 2.5, whereas another demonstrated a 2.4-fold increase in risk of SDH formation with increasing doses of dabigatran.[8,9] The impact of preoperative antithrombosis on hematoma recurrence postoperatively remains controversial.[10–15]

Patients on antithrombosis presenting with acute or chronic SDHs are thought to be at higher likelihood of presenting with larger hematomas or more severe neurologic deficits. Although the literature specific to SDH is limited on the impact of antithrombosis on hematoma size or propensity for expansion,[16] there is strong evidence for increased expansion of intracerebral hematomas (ICHs) with warfarin anticoagulation.[17,18] Standard neurosurgical and neurocritical care of subdural hematomas, therefore, involves reversal of antithrombosis preoperatively, where possible, and a

Disclosures: R.L. Macdonald is Chief Scientific Officer of Edge Therapeutics, Inc.
[a] Division of Neurosurgery, Department of Surgery, Toronto Western Hospital, University of Toronto, 399 Bathurst Street, West Wing, 4th Floor, Toronto, Ontario M5T 2S8, Canada; [b] Division of Neurosurgery, Keenan Research Centre for Biomedical Science, Li Ka Shing Knowledge Institute, St. Michael's Hospital, 30 Bond Street, Toronto, Ontario M5B 1W8, Canada
* Corresponding author. Division of Neurosurgery, St. Michael's Hospital, 30 Bond Street, Toronto, Ontario M5B 1W8, Canada.
E-mail address: macdonaldlo@smh.ca

Neurosurg Clin N Am 28 (2017) 287–295
http://dx.doi.org/10.1016/j.nec.2016.11.011
1042-3680/17/© 2016 Elsevier Inc. All rights reserved.

thorough individualized risk-benefit assessment of antithrombosis resumption.

This article highlights the spectrum of antithrombotic agents in common use, their mechanisms of action, and strategies for reversal. The current evidence for antithrombosis resumption, with available metrics for stratifying hemorrhagic and thromboembolic risk, is also reviewed.

PLATELET ACTIVATION

The initial response to endothelial injury begins with platelet adhesion to exposed extracellular matrix (**Fig. 1**). This interaction is mediated by the glycoprotein (GP) Ib/V/IX receptor complex on the platelet surface and von Willebrand factor bound to exposed collagen at the site of vessel injury. Adhesion leads to platelet activation by several pathways, initiated by collagen, ADP, thromboxane A_2, serotonin, and thrombin (factor II).[19] Collectively, these pathways alter the morphology as

well as secretory and receptor phenotypes of platelets into an active form. The primary effector of activated platelets is the GPIIb/IIIa surface receptor, activation of which is responsible for mediating platelet aggregation and thrombus propagation, stabilized by fibrin deposition from concurrent activation of coagulation cascades.[19]

COAGULATION CASCADE

Classically, the coagulation cascade comprises an extrinsic pathway, initiated by tissue injury, and a contact-initiated intrinsic pathway, both leading to a common final pathway (**Fig. 2**). This system is useful for understanding tests of coagulation activity but is likely simplified from current understanding of coagulation as a cell-based and surface-based process.[20] Prolonged activated partial thromboplastin time (aPTT) may be secondary to heparin; lupus anticoagulant; deficiencies of factors 8, 9, and 11; and von Willebrand disease.

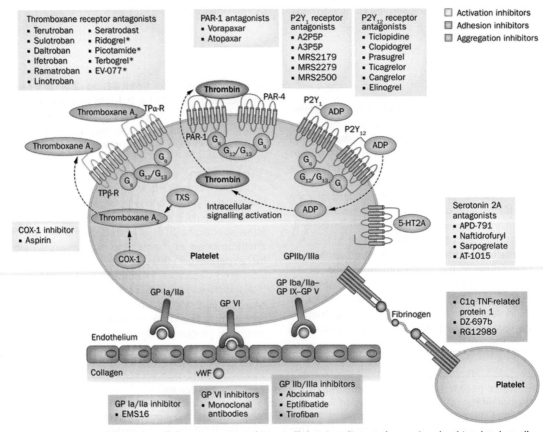

Fig. 1. A summary of the extracellular receptors and intracellular signaling pathways involved in platelet adherence to injured vascular endothelium, activation, and aggregation. Current and emerging drugs inhibiting platelet activation, adhesion, and aggregation are shown in boxes. 5-HT2A, serotonin receptor 2A; PAR, protease-activated receptor; TP, thromboxane prostanoid receptor; TXS, thromboxane A_2 synthase; vWF, von Willebrand factor; * combined thromboxane-receptor antagonists and TXS inhibitors. (*From* Franchi F, Angiolillo DJ. Novel antiplatelet agents in acute coronary syndrome. Nat Rev Cardiol 2015;12(1):30–47; with permission.)

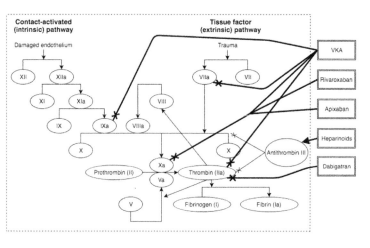

Fig. 2. A summary of the factors involved in the intrinsic and extrinsic coagulation cascades, culminating in the common pathway of the conversion of prothrombin (II) to thrombin (IIa). The factors potentiated (*arrowheads*) or inhibited (*X-arrowheads*) by common anticoagulant agents are shown.

An increased prothrombin time may be due to warfarin, vitamin K deficiency, liver dysfunction, or congenital factor 7 deficiency. Thrombin time depends on the conversion of fibrinogen to fibrin; hence, this test is sensitive to the detection of fibrinogen abnormalities and inhibitors acting at this level, such as heparin and dabigatran.

Fibrinolysis is initiated as a normal physiologic response for remodeling of a completed fibrin clot. It involves activation of plasminogens to plasmin by tissue and urokinase activators.[21] Fibrinolysis is inhibited endogenously by plasminogen activator inhibitor and thrombin-activatable fibrinolysis inhibitor, mainly α_2-antiplasmin. Exogenous inhibitors of fibrinolysis in current clinical use include aprotinin and the lysine derivatives tranexamic acid (TXA) and aminocaproic acid.

COMMON ANTIPLATELET AGENTS

A list of oral antiplatelet agents in common use, along with their relevant pharmacologic properties and reversal strategies, is shown in **Table 1**.

Current antiplatelet agents target predominantly 1 of 3 pathways. Acetylsalicylic acid (ASA) irreversibly inhibits cyclooxygenase (COX)-1 selectively (at low doses) or both COX-1 and COX-2 (at high doses), leading to anti-inflammatory and analgesic effects.[22] COX-1 inhibition attenuates the thromboxane A_2–mediated pathway of platelet activation (see **Fig. 1**).

Antagonists of the $P2Y_{12}$ receptor represent the second-most common class of antiplatelet drugs, including ticlopidine, clopidogrel, prasugrel, and ticagrelor, in order of their clinical development (see **Fig. 1**). Ticlopidine has largely been replaced by the latter agents because of its hematological side effects.[23] Clopidogrel and prasugrel, both thienopyridines, are active only in their metabolite

form and irreversibly bind the ADP binding site on the $P2Y_{12}$ receptor. Ticagrelor, a cyclopentyl-triazolo-pyrimidine, instead binds reversibly to a different site on the $P2Y_{12}$ receptor, thereby inhibiting G protein–coupled signaling, in both prodrug and metabolite forms (see **Fig. 1**).[22]

The GPIIb/IIIa inhibitors are commonly given intravenously (IV) in endovascular revascularization procedures. These are given intravascularly; there are no enteral formulations available. Agents in this class include abciximab, eptifibatide, and tirofiban.[24]

Reversal strategies for commonly prescribed antiplatelet drugs relate directly to their mechanism of action. Because both ASA and the thienopyridines (clopidogrel and prasugrel) bind irreversibly to their targets, transfusion of exogenous platelets beyond the circulating half-life of both drugs somewhat attenuates their effect, although full reversal requires turnover of the endogenous platelet pool, typically over 2 to 3 days.[25] A higher platelet transfusion mass seems to be required for thienopyridines than ASA.[26] By contrast, because ticagrelor binding is reversible, circulating ticagrelor and its metabolite likely inhibit exogenously introduced platelets as well, limiting the effectiveness of platelet transfusions.[27,28]

COMMON ANTICOAGULANT AGENTS

A list of anticoagulant agents in common use, along with their relevant pharmacologic properties and reversal strategies, is shown in **Table 2**.

Commonly prescribed anticoagulant drugs fall into 3 classes: heparin based, vitamin K antagonists (VKAs), and novel oral anticoagulants (NOACs). Unfractionated heparin (UFH) and low-molecular-weight heparins (LMWHs), including enoxaparin, dalteparin, and tinzaparin, potentiate

Table 1
Common oral antiplatelet agents

Generic Name	Mechanism of Action	Elimination Half-Life	Reversal Strategy	Laboratory Monitoring
ASA	Irreversible COX inhibition	20 min	Platelet transfusion (4–5 U); desmopressin (0.3 µg/kg IV)	Arachidonic acid–based testing (VerifyNow ASA)
Dipyridamole	Phosphodiesterase inhibitor	10–12 h	None	None
Ticlopidine	Thienopyridine — irreversible $P2Y_{12}$ receptor inhibition	4–5 d	None	Bleeding time
Clopidogrel	Thienopyridine — irreversible $P2Y_{12}$ receptor inhibition	6 h	Platelet transfusion (10 U q12 h × 48 h); desmopressin (0.3 µg/kg IV)	$P2Y_{12}$ receptor cascade test (VerifyNow $P2Y_{12}$)
Prasugrel	Thienopyridine — irreversible $P2Y_{12}$ receptor inhibition	2–15 h	Platelet transfusion (10 U q12 h × 48 h); desmopressin (0.3 µg/kg IV)	$P2Y_{12}$ receptor cascade test (VerifyNow $P2Y_{12}$)
Ticagrelor	Cyclopentyl-triazolo-pyrimidine — reversible $P2Y_{12}$ receptor inhibition	7 h	None	None

Table 2
Common oral anticoagulant agents

Generic Name	Mechanism of Action	Elimination Half-Life	Reversal Strategy	Laboratory Monitoring
Warfarin	Inhibition of hepatic production of vitamin K–dependent factors	T1/2: 25–60 h	Vitamin K 5–10 mg IV plus PCC at weight-based dosing (25–100 U/kg IV); FFP (15 mL/kg IV)	INR
Dabigatran	Direct thrombin (IIa) inhibition	T1/2: 12–14 h	Idarucizumab 5 g IV + 2.5 g IV (1 h apart); PCC (25–100 U/kg IV); FFP (15 mL/kg IV); rVIIa (10–90 µg/kg IV); hemodialysis	aPTT
Rivaroxaban	Factor Xa inhibition	T1/2: 7–11 h	PCC (25–100 U/kg IV); FFP (15 mL/kg IV); rVIIa (10–90 µg/kg IV)	Anti–factor Xa assay
Apixaban	Factor Xa inhibition	T1/2: 8–15 h	PCC (25–100 U/kg IV); FFP (15 mL/kg IV); rVIIa (10–90 µg/kg IV)	Anti–factor Xa assay

antithrombin III–mediated inhibition of factor Xa (see **Fig. 2**). UFH inhibits thrombin as well as factor Xa so its effect is detected in the aPTT whereas LMWHs inhibit factor Xa and generally do not affect the aPTT. UFH is administered either IV or subcutaneously, whereas LMWHs are typically given only subcutaneously.

Warfarin was the first drug of the VKA class. Warfarin interferes with the conversion of vitamin K to its 2,3 epoxide, inhibiting the activity of vitamin K–dependent procoagulant factors (factors II, VII, IX, and X) as well as reducing the anticoagulant activity of proteins C and S.[22,24]

NOACs are targeted inhibitors of either factor Xa or thrombin directly. Oral Xa inhibitors include rivaroxaban and apixaban, whereas fondaparinux is a subcutaneously administered Xa inhibitor. Rivaroxaban and apixaban reversibly bind the active site of free and bound Xa molecules, whereas fondaparinux achieves indirect Xa inhibition through interaction with antithrombin III. Direct thrombin inhibitors include argatroban and bivalirudin (parenteral) as well as dabigatran (oral). All function via direct, competitive inhibition of the thrombin active site, without requirement for cofactors; hence, their efficacy is reported to be less variable although monitoring of and reversal of their activities is more problematic (see **Fig. 2**).

Reversal of heparin-based drugs is accomplished by direct ionic interaction and binding of heparin to protamine, a cationic protein. Reversal of VKA is accomplished, in the acute phase, by direct replacement of vitamin K–dependent procoagulant factors and, in the subacute phase, with vitamin K replenishment. Due to their reversible binding, reversal of NOACs is considerably more variable, with only 1 specific agent receiving accelerated approval: idarucizumab, a humanized monoclonal antibody fragment that binds dabigatran. Replacement of factors from various sources, including fresh frozen plasma (FFP), cryoprecipitate, prothrombin complex concentrate (PCC), recombinant activated factor VII (rVIIa), and factor VIII inhibitor bypassing activity, has been attempted with varying efficacy.[29]

PREOPERATIVE MANAGEMENT OF ANTITHROMBOSIS

The initial management of a patient with an SDH who is taking anticoagulant or antiplatelet drugs involves standard medical stabilization and medical management of elevated intracranial pressure, if required. A thorough history should be obtained, where possible, of the type and dose of antithrombotic agent, the duration and indication for prescription, medical comorbidities, and additional medications that may alter antithrombotic metabolism as well as the timing of the last antithrombotic dose. Laboratory measurements should be obtained to adequately assess current antithrombotic activity. The appropriate tests for each class of antiplatelet and anticoagulant are shown in **Tables 1** and **2**, respectively.

A risk-benefit assessment should be performed for reversal of antithrombosis because there is limited high-level evidence to support emergency reversal of antiplatelet/anticoagulant drugs and such reversal is associated with risk of complications, including thrombosis, for which the patient was initially given these drugs. Consultation with other relevant medical and surgical specialties is frequently required. The anticoagulant or antiplatelet drug should usually be discontinued. In general, however, patients presenting in extremis warrant immediate preoperative reversal of antithrombosis, regardless of the indication for the drug. For all oral agents, a history of ingestion within 2 hours of presentation, although uncommon, particularly for loading doses or overdoses, merits consideration of the use of oral activated charcoal to promote absorption and reduce gastrointestinal bioavailability.[30]

Reversal of anticoagulant drugs in patients with ICH reduces the risk of expansion of the ICH, particularly for warfarin, although the effect on clinical outcome is less clear.[31] There are no randomized clinical trials and only few data on indications for reversal of anticoagulant agents in patients with acute or chronic SDH. Only general recommendations can be made, and the approach to these patients should be individualized. It is reasonable to emergently reverse anticoagulant drugs in patients who require emergency surgery for hematoma evacuation (altered consciousness, focal neurologic deficits, and so forth) or neuroimaging findings suggestive of the possibility of acute neurologic deterioration in situations where the risks are acceptable. The balance currently favors reversal of anticoagulation in a majority of patients with acute or chronic SDH.[32] On the other hand, highly risky therapeutic approaches to reverse anticoagulant drugs should generally be avoided unless there is strong evidence to support efficacy of the intervention, for example, in patients with acute life-threatening thrombosis, disseminated intravascular coagulation, or heparin-induced thrombocytopenia.[32]

A summary of available reversal methods for common anticoagulant drugs is shown in **Table 2**. For warfarin, fast-acting replacement of vitamin K–dependent coagulation factors is the mainstay of acute reversal. This may be accomplished by any of FFP, PCC, and rVIIa. FFP, however, requires a high-volume infusion and is deficient in factor IX; therefore, it is associated with higher rates of pulmonary edema and delayed international normalized ratio (INR) reversal.[29] rVIIa, although immediately effective for both INR reversal and at least radiographic stabilization of ICH volume (unknown for SDH), is associated with increased thromboembolic complications but not with improved outcome and, hence, should be avoided as a first-line reversal agent for anticoagulant-related ICH.[33,34] PCC, containing 3 (II, IX, and X) or 4 (II, VII, IX, and X) factors, is the fastest, most effective method of warfarin reversal, particularly when used with individualized dosing based on body weight and initial INR.[35,36] A target preoperative INR of 1.5 may be achieved within 15 minutes of infusion with weight-based dosing (see **Table 2**). IV vitamin K is typically administered concomitantly for prolonged anticoagulation reversal over the subsequent 24 hours.

Reversal of NOACs, although not as robustly associated with reduced ICH expansion as warfarin, should nonetheless be attempted. Available strategies are similar to those for warfarin; however, FFP, PCC, and/or rVIIa have shown poor efficacy for dabigatran and only moderate efficacy for rivaroxaban and apixaban.[37] Activated PCC has shown some in vitro efficacy for dabigatran, but this has not been replicated in clinical studies.[38] Dabigatran is cleared by the kidneys; hence, particularly in patients with preexisting renal dysfunction, hemodialysis may be considered to expedite clearance and prolong reversal of anticoagulation.[39] A novel monoclonal antibody fragment targeting unbound dabigatran, idarucizumab, has received accelerated approved for US clinical use as of October 2015, and likely represents the best available method of emergency dabigatran reversal.[40,41] PCC, at weight-based dosing (see **Table 2**), is the best available emergency reversal method for rivaroxaban and apixaban at present. Novel soluble decoy factors, however, such as andexanet alfa, are in development for the reversal of factor Xa inhibitors.[41,42]

Because reversal agents for all anticoagulant drugs differ in activity based on manufacturer, efficacy of reversal should be tested preoperatively with the appropriate laboratory metrics. The recommended laboratory tests for each anticoagulant are shown in **Table 2**.

Evidence supporting preoperative reversal of antiplatelet drugs is less convincing than for anticoagulants. Although some studies have associated increased platelet inhibition with increased ICH volume expansion and platelet transfusion within 12 hours of presentation with improved functional outcomes, others have shown no benefit with attempted reversal via platelet transfusion.[43–45] The lack of association between antiplatelet drugs and functional outcomes and the significant variability in laboratory testing of platelet function have created uncertainty in the efficacy and utility of antiplatelet reversal. Most of the data are derived from patients with ICH and there is no high-level evidence to guide management in patients with SDH. Whether extrapolating from ICH to SDH is appropriate is unknown. In a large randomized controlled trial of platelet transfusion in ICH patients on antiplatelet agents, platelet transfusion within 6 hours of presentation was associated with significantly worse functional outcomes and increased adverse events.[46] Current guidelines in the setting of antiplatelet-related ICH or SDH recommend discontinuing the antiplatelet agent but administering platelets only to patients who under neurosurgical intervention. Platelet transfusions are not recommended in patients who do not require neurosurgical intervention.[32] Desmopressin (DDAVP) has shown some promise in ICH and other types of intracranial hemorrhage at restoring platelet function and improving functional outcomes, albeit in smaller studies.[47,48] Given its minimal side-effect profile, current guidelines recommend the administration of 0.4 µg/kg IV of DDAVP for antiplatelet-related intracranial hemorrhage, which may be combined with platelet transfusion in patients undergoing surgery.[32] Although rVIIa and fibrinogen supplementation have been attempted in preclinical trials, neither has demonstrated sufficient benefit for recommendation.

INTRAOPERATIVE MANAGEMENT OF ANTITHROMBOSIS

The use of antifibrinolytic agents, most commonly TXA, has been studied extensively for minimization of intraoperative blood loss. In the trauma literature, intraoperative TXA administration has proved effective to reduce bleeding-related mortality.[49] Although no high-level evidence for preoperative or intraoperative TXA exists in neurosurgery, administration of TXA in conservatively managed chronic SDH has been reported and is under further investigation in randomized trials.[50–52] Given the prothrombotic and epileptogenic risks of TXA, widespread adoption of TXA for chronic SDH should await the results of these studies.[53,54] Otherwise, ongoing surgical bleeding is most often the result of inadequate surgical technique rather than previously undiagnosed bleeding diatheses. Treatment should be guided by clinical suspicions and laboratory tests.

POSTOPERATIVE RESUMPTION OF ANTITHROMBOSIS

Patients on anticoagulant and antiplatelet drugs are at higher risk for the development of chronic SDH and larger acute SDH with greater severity at presentation. Preoperative antithrombosis, however, has not been as clearly associated with postoperative recurrence in the literature, although retrospective analyses for chronic SDH reveal up to a 33% recurrence rate for patients on antithrombosis versus up to 15% for patients not taking these drugs.[6] One study found an almost 2-fold increased risk of rebleeding after surgical evacuation of chronic SDH in patients who were on aspirin or warfarin preoperatively but not in patients on clopidogrel.[55]

Resumption of antithrombosis postoperatively requires balancing the risks of rebleeding with the risks of thromboembolic complications if antithrombotics are not resumed. Almost all data regarding restarting antithrombotics in patients with SDH are retrospective and not from well-controlled prospective studies or randomized trials. Although there is limited high-level evidence to guide resumption of antithrombosis after evacuation of subdural hematomas, there is some literature pertaining to chronic SDH that suggests that early resumption, at 72 hours postoperatively, may be safe. In patients with mechanical valves, warfarin resumption at 3 to 5 days postevacuation of chronic SDH did not increase the risk of subsequent recurrence.[12,56–58] Resumption of antiplatelet agents 1 week after chronic SDH evacuation has also been reported, with no increase in subsequent recurrence.[15] In a retrospective series of surgically managed chronic SDH, thromboembolic complications in anticoagulated patients peaked at 3 days postoperatively, with no increase in recurrence risk when antithrombosis was resumed; hence, resumption at 3 days may be safe.[55] Unfortunately, the literature on the resumption of newer oral anticoagulants after SDH evacuation remains bare.

Ultimately, whether and when to resume antithrombosis postoperatively must be decided on an individualized basis, with the assistance of medical and hematologic subspecialties for risk stratification. Where available, validated objective grading systems should be used to quantitate risk.[59] For thrombotic risk, these include the CHA_2DS_2-VASc in atrial fibrillation; for hemorrhagic risk, these include the $HEMORR_2HAGES$, HAS-BLED, and ATRIA scores.[60–62] Review of such data, for example, may indicate that in some cases the risk of thromboembolic complications, such as in elderly chronic SDH patients with atrial fibrillation and a low CHA_2DS_2-VASc score, may exceed the benefits.

SUMMARY

- Antithrombosis should be reversed emergently in all surgical SDH patients presenting in extremis.
- Warfarin should be reversed with 3-factor PCC or activated PCC, with concomitant vitamin K.
- Idarucizumab should be considered for reversal of dabigatran.
- Activated PCC is the best reversal option for factor Xa inhibitors.
- There is no strong evidence to support platelet transfusions for the reversal of antiplatelet drugs, although this is recommended in patients who require neurosurgical operations.
- Desmopressin may be considered for reversal of antiplatelet agents, acknowledging its limited efficacy.
- Appropriate laboratory monitoring should guide the adequacy of reversal for all agents.
- Postoperative resumption of antithrombosis should be guided by an individualized assessment of hemorrhagic and thromboembolic risk.

REFERENCES

1. Fuster V, Mearns BM. The CVD paradox: mortality vs prevalence. Nat Rev Cardiol 2009;6(11):669.
2. Go AS, Hylek EM, Phillips KA, et al. Prevalence of diagnosed atrial fibrillation in adults: national implications for rhythm management and stroke prevention: the AnTicoagulation and Risk Factors in Atrial Fibrillation (ATRIA) Study. JAMA 2001;285(18): 2370–5.
3. Rogacka R, Chieffo A, Michev I, et al. Dual antiplatelet therapy after percutaneous coronary intervention with stent implantation in patients taking chronic oral anticoagulation. JACC Cardiovasc Interv 2008;1(1): 56–61.
4. Lièvre M, Cucherat M. Aspirin in the secondary prevention of cardiovascular disease: an update of the APTC meta-analysis. Fundam Clin Pharmacol 2010; 24(3):385–91.
5. Connolly S, Pogue J, Hart R, et al. Clopidogrel plus aspirin versus oral anticoagulation for atrial fibrillation in the Atrial fibrillation Clopidogrel Trial with Irbesartan for prevention of Vascular Events (ACTIVE W): a randomised controlled trial. Lancet 2006; 367(9526):1903–12.
6. Ducruet AF, Grobelny BT, Zacharia BE, et al. The surgical management of chronic subdural hematoma. Neurosurg Rev 2012;35(2):155–69.

7. Reymond MA, Marbet G, Radü EW, et al. Aspirin as a risk factor for hemorrhage in patients with head injuries. Neurosurg Rev 1992;15(1):21–5. Available at: http://www.ncbi.nlm.nih.gov/pubmed/1584433. Accessed June 28, 2016.

8. Hylek EM, Singer DE. Risk factors for intracranial hemorrhage in outpatients taking warfarin. Ann Intern Med 1994;120(11):897–902. Available at: http://www.ncbi.nlm.nih.gov/pubmed/8172435. Accessed June 28, 2016.

9. Hart RG, Diener H-C, Yang S, et al. Intracranial hemorrhage in atrial fibrillation patients during anticoagulation with warfarin or dabigatran: the RE-LY trial. Stroke 2012;43(6):1511–7.

10. Chon K-H, Lee J-M, Koh E-J, et al. Independent predictors for recurrence of chronic subdural hematoma. Acta Neurochir 2012;154:1541–8.

11. Forster MT, Mathe AK, Senft C, et al. The influence of preoperative anticoagulation on outcome and quality of life after surgical treatment of chronic subdural hematoma. J Clin Neurosci 2010;17(8):975–9.

12. Gonugunta V, Buxton N. Warfarin and chronic subdural haematomas. Br J Neurosurg 2001;15(6):514–7.

13. Rust T, Kiemer N, Erasmus A. Chronic subdural haematomas and anticoagulation or anti-thrombotic therapy. J Clin Neurosci 2006;13(8):823–7.

14. Stanisic M, Lund-Johansen M, Mahesparan R. Treatment of chronic subdural hematoma by burr-hole craniostomy in adults: influence of some factors on postoperative recurrence. Acta Neurochir 2005; 147:1249–56.

15. Torihashi K, Sadamasa N, Yoshida K, et al. Independent predictors for recurrence of chronic subdural hematoma: a review of 343 consecutive surgical cases. Neurosurgery 2008;63:1125–9.

16. Szczygielski J, Gund S-M, Schwerdtfeger K, et al. Factors affecting outcome in treatment of chronic subdural hematoma in ICU patients: impact of anticoagulation. World Neurosurg 2016;92:426–33.

17. Purrucker JC, Haas K, Rizos T, et al. Early clinical and radiological course, management, and outcome of intracerebral hemorrhage related to new oral anticoagulants. JAMA Neurol 2016;73(2):169.

18. Huynh TJ, Aviv RI, Dowlatshahi D, et al. Validation of the 9-Point and 24-Point hematoma expansion prediction scores and derivation of the PREDICT A/B scores. Stroke 2015;46(11):3105–10.

19. Jennings L. Mechanisms of platelet activation: need for new strategies to protect against platelet-mediated atherothrombosis. Thromb Haemost 2009;102(2):248–57.

20. Versteeg HH, Heemskerk JW, Levi M, et al. New fundamentals in hemostasis. Physiol Rev 2013;93(1): 327–58.

21. Rijken DC, Lijnen HR. New insights into the molecular mechanisms of the fibrinolytic system. J Thromb Haemost 2009;7(1):4–13.

22. Mega JL, Simon T. Pharmacology of antithrombotic drugs: an assessment of oral antiplatelet and anticoagulant treatments. Lancet 2015;386(9990):281–91.

23. Bertrand M, Rupprecht H, Urban P, et al. Double-blind study of the safety of clopidogrel with and without a loading dose in combination with aspirin compared with ticlopidine in combination with aspirin after coronary stenting: the clopidogrel aspirin stent international cooperative study. Circulation 2000;102(6):624–9.

24. Yorkgitis BK, Ruggia-Check C, Dujon JE. Antiplatelet and anticoagulation medications and the surgical patient. Am J Surg 2014;207(1):95–101.

25. Awtry EH, Loscalzo J. Aspirin. Circulation 2000; 101(10):1206–18.

26. Vilahur G, Choi BG, Zafar MU, et al. Normalization of platelet reactivity in clopidogrel-treated subjects. J Thromb Haemost 2007;5(1):82–90.

27. Sugidachi A, Ohno K, Ogawa T, et al. A comparison of the pharmacological profiles of prasugrel and ticagrelor assessed by platelet aggregation, thrombus formation and haemostasis in rats. Br J Pharmacol 2013;169(1):82–9.

28. Godier A, Taylor G, Gaussem P. Inefficacy of platelet transfusion to reverse ticagrelor. N Engl J Med 2015; 372(2):196–7.

29. Mittal MK, Rabinstein AA. Anticoagulation-related intracranial hemorrhages. Curr Atheroscler Rep 2012;14(4):351–9.

30. James RF, Palys V, Lomboy JR, et al. The role of anticoagulants, antiplatelet agents, and their reversal strategies in the management of intracerebral hemorrhage. Neurosurg Focus 2013;34(5):E6.

31. Huttner HB, Schellinger PD, Hartmann M, et al. Hematoma growth and outcome in treated neurocritical care patients with intracerebral hemorrhage related to oral anticoagulant therapy: comparison of acute treatment strategies using vitamin K, fresh frozen plasma, and prothrombin complex concentrates. Stroke 2006;37(6):1465–70.

32. Frontera JA, Lewin JJ III, Rabinstein AA, et al. Guideline for Reversal of antithrombotics in intracranial hemorrhage. Neurocrit Care 2016;24(1): 6–46.

33. Mayer SA, Brun NC, Begtrup K, et al. Efficacy and safety of recombinant activated factor VII for acute intracerebral hemorrhage. N Engl J Med 2008; 358(20):2127–37.

34. Yuan ZH, Jiang JK, Huang WD, et al. A meta-analysis of the efficacy and safety of recombinant activated factor VII for patients with acute intracerebral hemorrhage without hemophilia. J Clin Neurosci 2010;17(6):685–93.

35. van Aart L, Eijkhout HW, Kamphuis JS, et al. Individualized dosing regimen for prothrombin complex concentrate more effective than standard treatment in the reversal of oral anticoagulant therapy: an

open, prospective randomized controlled trial. Thromb Res 2006;118(3):313–20.

36. Guest JF, Watson HG, Limaye S. Modeling the cost-effectiveness of prothrombin complex concentrate compared with fresh frozen plasma in emergency warfarin reversal in the United Kingdom. Clin Ther 2010;32(14):2478–93.

37. Eerenberg ES, Kamphuisen PW, Sijpkens MK, et al. Reversal of rivaroxaban and dabigatran by pro-thrombin complex concentrate: a randomized, placebo-controlled, crossover study in healthy sub-jects. Circulation 2011;124(14):1573–9.

38. Lindahl TL, Wallstedt M, Gustafsson KM, et al. More efficient reversal of dabigatran inhibition of coagula-tion by activated prothrombin complex concentrate or recombinant factor VIIa than by four-factor pro-thrombin complex concentrate. Thromb Res 2015; 135(3):544–7.

39. Stangier J, Rathgen K, Stähle H, et al. Influence of renal impairment on the pharmacokinetics and phar-macodynamics of oral dabigatran etexilate. Clin Pharmacokinet 2010;49(4):259–68.

40. Glund S, Stangier J, Schmohl M, et al. Safety, toler-ability, and efficacy of idarucizumab for the reversal of the anticoagulant effect of dabigatran in healthy male volunteers: a randomised, placebo-controlled, double-blind phase 1 trial. Lancet 2015; 386(9994):680–90.

41. Smythe MA, Trujillo T, Fanikos J. Reversal agents for use with direct and indirect anticoagulants. Am J Health Syst Pharm 2016;73(10 Supplement 2):S27–48.

42. Hu TY, Vaidya VR, Asirvatham SJ. Reversing antico-agulant effects of novel oral anticoagulants: role of ciraparantag, andexanet alfa, and idarucizumab. Vasc Health Risk Manag 2016;12:35–44.

43. Ducruet AF, Hickman ZL, Zacharia BE, et al. Impact of platelet transfusion on hematoma expansion in patients receiving antiplatelet agents before intrace-rebral hemorrhage. Neurol Res 2010;32(7):706–10.

44. Naidech AM, Liebling SM, Rosenberg NF, et al. Early platelet transfusion improves platelet activity and may improve outcomes after intracerebral hemor-rhage. Neurocrit Care 2012;16(1):82–7.

45. Naidech AM, Bendok BR, Garg RK, et al. Reduced platelet activity is associated with more intraventric-ular hemorrhage. Neurosurgery 2009;65(4):684–8 [discussion: 688].

46. Baharoglu MI, Cordonnier C, Salman RA-S, et al. Platelet transfusion versus standard care after acute stroke due to spontaneous cerebral haemorrhage associated with antiplatelet therapy (PATCH): a randomised, open-label, phase 3 trial. Lancet 2016;387(10038):2605–13.

47. Naidech AM, Maas MB, Levasseur-Franklin KE, et al. Desmopressin improves platelet activity in acute intracerebral hemorrhage. Stroke 2014;45(8): 2451–3.

48. Kapapa T, Röhrer S, Struve S, et al. Desmopressin acetate in intracranial haemorrhage. Neurol Res Int 2014;2014:298767.

49. Roberts I, Shakur H, Coats T, et al. The CRASH-2 trial: a randomised controlled trial and economic evaluation of the effects of tranexamic acid on death, vascular occlusive events and transfusion requirement in bleeding trauma patients. Health Technol Assess 2013;17(10):1–79.

50. Kageyama H, Toyooka T, Tsuzuki N, et al. Nonsur-gical treatment of chronic subdural hematoma with tranexamic acid. J Neurosurg 2013;119(2):332–7.

51. Tanweer O, Frisoli FA, Bravate C, et al. Tranexamic acid for treatment of residual subdural hematoma af-ter bedside twist-drill evacuation. World Neurosurg 2016;91:29–33.

52. Iorio-Morin C, Blanchard J, Richer M, et al. Tranexa-mic Acid in Chronic Subdural Hematomas (TRACS): study protocol for a randomized controlled trial. Tri-als 2016;17(1):235.

53. Lecker I, Wang D-S, Romaschin AD, et al. Tranexa-mic acid concentrations associated with human sei-zures inhibit glycine receptors. J Clin Invest 2012; 122(12):4654–66.

54. Meier K, Hoesch R. Antifibrinolytic therapy in intracra-nial hemorrhage. Drug Dev Res 2013;74(7):478–84.

55. Guha D, Coyne S, Macdonald RL. Timing of the resumption of antithrombotic agents following surgi-cal evacuation of chronic subdural hematomas: a retrospective cohort study. J Neurosurg 2016; 124(3):750–9.

56. Chari A, Clemente Morgado T, Rigamonti D. Recom-mencement of anticoagulation in chronic subdural haematoma: a systematic review and meta-analysis. Br J Neurosurg 2014;28(1):2–7.

57. Kawamata T, Takeshita M, Kubo O, et al. Manage-ment of intracranial hemorrhage associated with anti-coagulant therapy. Surg Neurol 1995;44(5):438–42.

58. Yeon JY, Kong DS, Hong SC. Safety of early warfarin resumption following burr hole drainage for warfarin-associated subacute or chronic subdural hemor-rhage. J Neurotrauma 2012;29(7):1334–41.

59. Lane DA, Lip GYH. Use of the CHA2DS2-VASc and HAS-BLED Scores to Aid Decision Making for Thromboprophylaxis in Nonvalvular Atrial Fibrillation. Circulation 2012;126(7):860–5.

60. Gage BF, Yan Y, Milligan PE, et al. Clinical classifica-tion schemes for predicting hemorrhage: results from the National Registry of Atrial Fibrillation (NRAF). Am Heart J 2006;151(3):713–9.

61. Pisters R, Lane DA, Nieuwlaat R, et al. A novel user-friendly score (HAS-BLED) to assess 1-year risk of major bleeding in patients with atrial fibrillation: the euro heart survey. Chest 2010;138(5):1093–100.

62. Fang MC, Go AS, Chang Y, et al. A new risk scheme to predict warfarin-associated hemorrhage. J Am Coll Cardiol 2011;58(4):395–401.

Index

Note: Page numbers of article titles are in **boldface** type.

Neurosurg Clin N Am 28 (2017) 297–300
http://dx.doi.org/10.1016/S1042-3680(17)30009-8
1042-3680/17

neurosurgery.theclinics.com

Moving?

Make sure your subscription moves with you!

To notify us of your new address, find your **Clinics Account Number** (located on your mailing label above your name), and contact customer service at:

Email: journalscustomerservice-usa@elsevier.com

800-654-2452 (subscribers in the U.S. & Canada)
314-447-8871 (subscribers outside of the U.S. & Canada)

Fax number: 314-447-8029

Elsevier Health Sciences Division
Subscription Customer Service
3251 Riverport Lane
Maryland Heights, MO 63043

Printed and bound by CPI Group (UK) Ltd, Croydon, CR0 4YY

08/05/2025

01864699-0015